LECTURES IN PSYCHIATRY

LECTURES IN PSYCHIATRY

THE FUNCTIONAL PSYCHOSES:

The Schizophrenias and Major Affective Disorders

by

KEN REED, Ph.D., M.D.

Department of Psychiatry and Behavioral Sciences

The University of Texas Health Science Center Houston, Texas

WARREN H. GREEN, INC.
St. Louis, Missouri, U. S. A.

Published by

WARREN H. GREEN, INC.
8356 Olive Blvd.
St. Louis, Missouri 63132, U.S.A.

ISBN No. 0-87527-339-4

Printed in the United States of America

PREFACE

This book is based on a series of lectures that I give to senior medical students during their clinical rotation in psychiatry. It was written at their suggestion with their needs specifically in mind. Hopefully it will prove useful to other clinicians involved with the care of patients with these disorders. This book is not intended as a reference text, but perhaps it may stimulate some students to read the definitive books and papers.

Ken Reed Ph.D., M.D.

Houston, 1985

CONTENTS

LECTURES IN PSYCHIATRY

CHAPTER 1

INTRODUCTION

In order to discuss "psychoses" it is first necessary to outline the concept of *mental state* which involves five components. These are *cognition, perception, affect, mobility* and *behaviour*. Each component will be defined in more detail later in the text but for now the layman's or dictionary concept of each term is adequate.

Each component in the mental state is influenced by the others. For example, perception is dependent on cognition, affect, mobility and behaviour and its evaluation of the same phenomena will differ as the other components vary. The interaction of these components normally involves *congruent* changes. For instance, if a poisonous snake is seen, one cognitively decides that there is a state of danger, the affect is fear and mobility and behaviour facilitate retreat.

There is normally *internal consistency* among the processes of a given component. The cognitive units which are involved in thinking through a problem have to "gel together." If one unit "does not compute," it is identified as internally inconsistent by the other cognitive units and rejected.

mental state
- cognition
- perception
- affect
- mobility
- behaviour

Figure 1

Mental disorders occur when the mental state is disturbed. The symptoms can be ascribed to perturbation of some component within the mental state. In general terms, the psychoses are mental disorders characterised by particular symptoms such as hallucinations from a disturbance of perception or delusions related to a perturbation of cognition.

It is crucial to realise that these symptoms can be caused by a variety of organic factors. Infections, toxins, metabolic disorders and trauma can all produce these symptoms as part of an *organic psychosis*. The psychotic disorders for which no organic etiology is demonstrable at our present level of knowledge are called *functional psychoses*.

These are no *pathognomonic* mental symptoms which differentiate the organic from the functional psychoses. All the symptoms seen in functional psychoses have occurred in organic psychoses. The memory deficits and disorientation characteristic of the organic psychoses can be mimicked by the symptoms of functional disorders. Therefore, it is not a simple matter to separate the two major psychotic groups.

The functional psychoses can be divided into two major categories, namely the *affective disorders* and the *schizophrenias*. This division is based on empirical data such as differences in lifetime course and outcome. Many of the same symptoms occur in both major categories of the func-

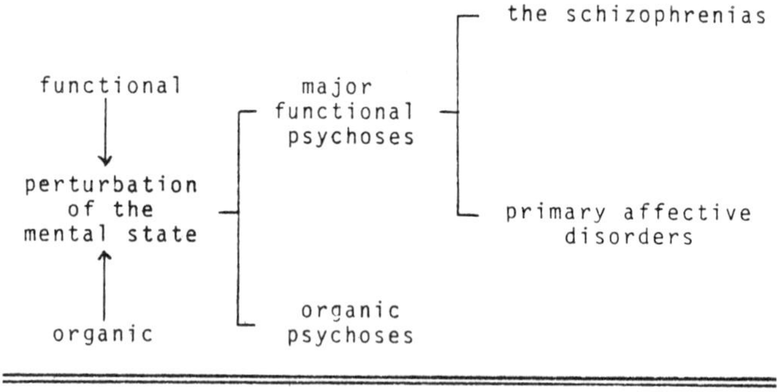

Figure 2

tional psychoses and there is no pathognomonic symptom which differentiates the two disorders.

The clinical syndromes of the psychoses, whether organic or functional in etiology, have a spectrum of symptoms with areas of commonality and overlap. This is schematically represented in the following figure.

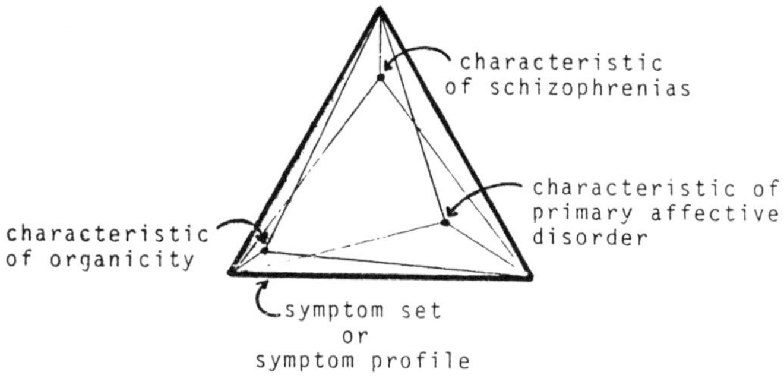

Figure 3

By definition, the organic psychoses produce symptoms as a result of demonstrable impairment of brain function. The major affective disorders have as their principal perturbation of the mental state the affect component.

The major affective disorders are:

> A group of mental disorders characterised by symptoms which reflect problems in cognition, perception, affect, mobility and behaviour relating to a perturbation of affect. Usually a prominent feature of the mental state is a disturbance of mood.

In the major affective disorders, the symptoms arising from a disturbance of components such as cognition or perception reflect an "extension" of the affect disturbance within the mental state.

The schizophrenias are:

> A group of mental disorders characterised by symptoms which reflect problems in cognition, perception, affect, mobility and behaviour. Excluded are those disorders whose symptoms are due to a core disturbance of affect or to demonstrable organic etiology.

Therefore, the diagnosis of a functional psychosis requires working through the differential diagnosis of an impaired mental state and demonstrating the fundamental features of the disorder. The possible toxic-organic etiologies for a patient's impaired mental state must be investigated, and, if identified, quickly treated.

The differentiation between the major functional psychoses is aided by additional information such as the patient's developmental history, family history of psychiatric disorders, and details of any previous psychiatric disorders including symptoms, course and response to treatment. This type of data is significantly different for the major affective disorders and the schizophrenias. Data of this type is equally useful in the diagnosis of non-psychiatric medical disorders.

CHAPTER 2

PSYCHOPATHOLOGY OF THE SCHIZOPHRENIAS

THE PSYCHOPATHOLOGY OF COGNITION

> Cognition is that operation of the mind by which one becomes aware of objects of thought and perception. It includes the processes of understanding and reason.

A particular train of thought or *cognitive set* can be represented as a series of linkages or *associations*. This cognitive set is a single option from a vast number which are in process at any given point in time.

The associations which occur within a set are subjected to *internal constraints* to ensure internal consistency. Consider the cognitive set, "John is Peter's brother; therefore, Peter is John's brother." This satisfies the normal constraints which result in *logical reasoning*. The cognition as a whole "accepts" this particular set and processes it as logical. In addition, this would be the case for anyone given the same data and circumstances.

On the other hand, the cognitive set, "The Virgin Mary is a woman, I am a woman; therefore, I am the Virgin Mary" violates normal internal constraints. In a non-perturbed cognition, this violation is recognised as "not computing" with the other cognitive sets and it is rejected.

The cognitive problem in schizophrenia is a pathological *loosening of association* which results in a lessening of internal constraints. In schizophrenia, the second cognitive set is not rejected by the overall cognition but is processed as being logical and acted upon.

The coexistence of pathological and non-pathological sets within the cognitive component is a salient feature of schizophrenia. To the schizophrenic, the second set is as "logical" as the first. The internal consistency of his reasoning is maintained and furthermore the other components of the mental state (perception, affect, mobility and behaviour) will process and respond to both sets equally.

It is redundant to ask if the schizophrenic thinks that the second set "makes sense" because as a result of the loosening of associations no discrepancies arise within his mental state.

An additional requirement for carrying through a logical train of thought is that cognitive sets which are extraneous to the task at hand be "filtered out." In schizophrenia, it is proposed that the internal filter is impaired. The result is a *failure to hold a single cognitive set* with the result that the thinking becomes *overinclusive* with an *interpenetration of themes*. Once again, this pathological process is not recognised as such by the other cognitive sets and the material which results is processed as logical.

These two models of schizophrenia can be applied to the organic psychoses and the affective disorders. In the former group, toxins such as amphetamines and alcohol or metabolic disorders such as hypothyroidism produce a loosening of associations and failure to hold a cognitive set by impairing brain function. In the affective disorders such as *manic-depressive psychoses* with cognitive psychopathology, the central affective disturbance has invaded cognition to cause a similar situation.

The symptoms of a *formal thought disorder* are reflected in large part by the schizophrenic's speech. This loses its communicative value since the sequence of pathological associations is known only to the patient and no apparent rhyme or reason for the linkage can be ascertained by the listener. Characteristic examples of the schizophrenic thought disorder are shown in the following figure which combines the two previously discussed models.

Speech may progress in a goal-oriented manner and suddenly become *tangential* for reasons unknown to the listener.

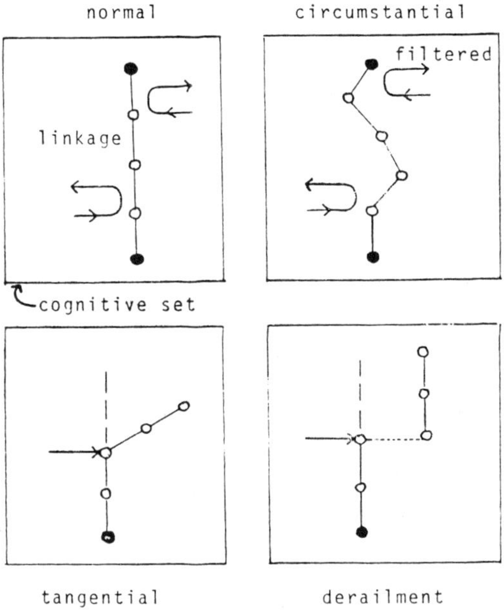

Figuire 4

More characteristically the speech becomes "like a river overflowing its banks." Rather than merely going off on a tangent, the speech *derails* to a new topic in no way related to the original set. In these cases the initial goal is never reached and the listener is aware of a "bizarre" quality in the shizophrenic's communication. This is in contrast to the milder non-psychotic speech characteristics of *circumstantionality* where the initial goal is eventually reached though by a circuitous route.

The schizophrenic may display *metonomy* in which a commonplace word is given significance understood only by the patient. More characteristically the patient uses a *neologism*, which is a word coined by the patient. It is often a condensation of words or themes known only to the patient. In the extreme case, the schizophrenic's speech takes on features of a *word salad* and loses all comprehensibility to others.

The severity of the thought disorder and associated peculiarities of speech depend on the degree of cognitive perturbation. In many cases, the formal thought disorder is subtle and easily overlooked in the background of normal cognitive sets. Patients displaying a word salad are rare and ought to be considered initially as having organic rather than functional psychoses. The vast majority of schizophrenic patients have pathological sets which are only a small fraction of the total cognitive processes. As a result, it should not be too surprising to find that a schizophrenic may still function at his job despite its requiring complex thought processes.

Since a formal thought disorder can lead to distractability and can impair concentration, it is possible that a schizophrenic will perform poorly on psychometric tests which evaluate intellectual functioning. Low scores in such tests should not be taken to mean that schizophrenia causes a primary dementia.

A second frequently seen feature of schizophrenia is a *delusion*. It must be stressed that although a delusion indicates a psychosis it is not definitive of schizophrenia or even of a functional disorder. A delusion is defined as a conviction resulting from a pathological cognitive set.

It is more than a belief which involves some degree of faith such as a belief in God or an "afterlife." A delusion is held with conviction, since the pathological set from which it is derived is not recognised as such by the patient's other cognitive processes. As a result of this internal consistency, the schizophrenic cannot be "talked out of it" any more than he can be persuaded by logical reasoning that a ball placed on a simple incline will roll upwards as opposed to downwards.

The delusion is idiosyncratic by virtue of being the product of a unique cognitive set whose processes are known and available only to that particular individual. If the *form* of the reasoning giving rise to the delusion is explained by the patient then it will be recognised as illogical by others, including other schizophrenics.

In the majority of cases, what is held with conviction, that is to say the *content* of the delusion, is clearly false. However, the crucial point regarding delusions is not what is held with conviction but rather the manner in which it was derived "logically" by the patient. It is wrong to assume that content which is eccentric, peculiar, different or simply false constitutes a delusion. Such a misusage changes the term delusion from referring to psychopathology and mental disorders to one of sociopathology and cultural norms. In fact, the content of a delusion which has been derived from a pathological cognitive set can be true. These points indicate the problems which can arise from the unnecessary use of the term false in defining a delusion.

As an illustration, consider the patient who presents with an unshakable conviction that his neighbours are plotting his downfall. This situation may have existed for many months and the patient's subsequent responses and behaviour may well cause his neighbors to be hostile and overly aggressive towards him. The result is that the delusion is subjected to a great deal of *secondary verification* which reenforces by non-pathological reasoning the pathologically derived conviction.

When the patient presents, he may explain the situation in terms of this secondary material and other neighbours and friends may vouch for the validity of the story. The crucial point is not what the man is convinced of but how he reasoned the situation through and what was the form of the original delusion event. Unfortunately, if the system has been developing over a prolonged time it may be very difficult to obtain the original pathological formation of the delusion. In acute cases, it is usually elicitable in the form of a *delusional perception.*

The key to a delusional conviction is the initial delusional perception which can be illustrated in the following manner. A schizophrenic is looking at a pipe lying in the ash tray on his desk. His perception of the items is absolutely normal and "he sees them as they are." The pathological step is that his set of normal perceptions will be processed by a cognitive component which has both pathological and non-pathological sets which coexist with internal consistency. This *two-memberedness* of the schizophrenic cognition is schematically shown in the following figure.

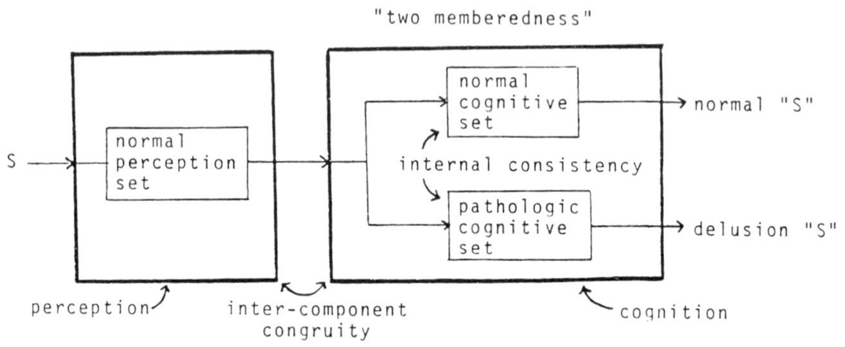

Figure 5

On the one hand, the normal perception set is processed by a logical cognitive set and is "understood for what it is." Simultaneously the same normal perception set is processed by a pathological cognitive set resulting in a pathological meaning. Because of the loosening of associations, these two interpretations are able to coexist with internal consistency and both will be processed as logical by the other components of the mental state. He reports "I knew it was simply my pipe in my ashtray, there was nothing unusual about it, but at the same time I *just knew* that it meant I was about to be assassinated." He says "I just knew it, it came to me in a flash, like a sign, I just knew it meant that."

This occurrence may be in the form of a *delusional idea.* A whole series of pathological convictions may crystallise at one time. Many things that the patient found puzzling "suddenly make sense now, as if the scales had fallen from my eyes."

As illustration of a delusional perception whose content is correct, consider a physician with an acute schizophrenic breakdown. The delusional content refers to him being a physician but he derives this not on the reasoning of clinical skills, training and privileges but "because of the way that the planes have changed their flight paths to come over my house." The delusional perception dominates and he says, "Look — I now know that the ultimate proof of my profession is not the medical school stuff but the planes. It suddenly came to me that that was the key." The content which refers to his being a physician is true but the form is based on pathological reasoning and represents the psychotic state.

It may be the delusional conviction is the only symptom of the psychosis at the time of presentation. Furthermore, his medical colleagues say that he was working fine up until they last saw him the previous evening. His wife says all was well except he had looked tired and preoccupied during the previous week.

The most common form of schizophrenic delusions is persecutory. Other types include grandiose, somatic, religious and erotic preoccupation and reasoning, for example, in the preceding order having discovered perpetual motion; having a body riddled with cancer; having been directly chosen by God to save the world; or having been passionately adored by a movie star. There is some degree of overlap in that having been chosen to save the world has features of grandiosity and possible persecution as well as religion. Erotic delusions are generally grandiose as well.

Once the primary delusion has been planted in the patient's mind a number of possibilities exist. The most benign is that the delusion will be *contained* or "walled off" with little effect on the overall functioning. Under such conditions, the patient will function at his premorbid level and will only become disturbed if the delusion is directly investigated.

Complete containment is rare and usually the delusional material undergoes some degree of *systematisation* within the mental state. This may involve inclusion of material which seems to be secondary verification with the result that the delusion becomes *incorporated* into the patient's lifestyle as a persistent and perhaps dominant theme. It should be noted this situation can have a morbidity for others than the schizophrenic. The family and acquaintances with whom he interacts are subjected to the delusional material and are an influence on the system.

The systematisation is added to by *ideas of reference*. This involves neutral events being given a personalised significance by the pathological cognitive sets. A schizophrenic with persecutory delusions may reason that his neighbours are plotting his demise when in fact they are simply in a group discussing the weather.

The delusional system may pervade the cognitive component, giving rise to a thought disorder. The resulting communication problems can further contribute to the development of the delusional pathology by incorporation.

The most common word used in discussions of delusions is *paranoid*. This word is used in everyday language as the description of a particular personality type. The paranoid personality is characterised by suspiciousness and a tendency to handle personal problems by ascribing them to the persecutory attitude and behaviour of others. This aspect of paranoid is widely employed in the medical setting.

The use of the word paranoid has had a chequered career with varied meanings. The initial use simply meant "out of one's mind" in the sense of "crazy" and so was a general term for the mentally disturbed person. The correct current usage is to indicate the presence of a primary delusion. This can have a number of types or forms with the most common being persecutory. The term *paranoid schizophrenia* implies a primary delusion but does not specify the nature of its content or form.

A *paranoid state* implies impaired mental functioning which gives rise to a primary delusion. The etiology may be toxic-organic or functional. If the disorder is a functional psychosis, then it can be schizophrenia or an affective disorder. A paranoid state requires the consideration of a wide differential diagnosis.

THE PSYCHOPATHOLOGY OF PERCEPTION

Perception is the conscious subjective awareness of objects and events in the environment (exteroception) and in one's body (interoception).

In schizophrenia, the perception component of the mental state consists of both pathological and non-pathological *perceptual sets*. These two types of sets coexist within the perception component with internal consistency.

The pathological perceptual sets make up only a small fraction of the total perceptual processes which are available. The product of a pathological set is not internally rejected by the non-pathological sets as being "invalid." The schizophrenic's "unreal" perceptions are as resistant to reasoning and logic as are delusions.

The occurence of an *hallucination* is indicative of a psychosis, but it is of little value in determining whether the etiology is organic or functional. An hallucination is symptomatic of a perturbation of perception and is defined as the registration of a perception in the absence of a stimulus.

In schizophrenia, the most common hallucinations are auditory. Other forms such as visual, tactile or olfactory occur in schizophrenia but tend to be accompanied by audi-

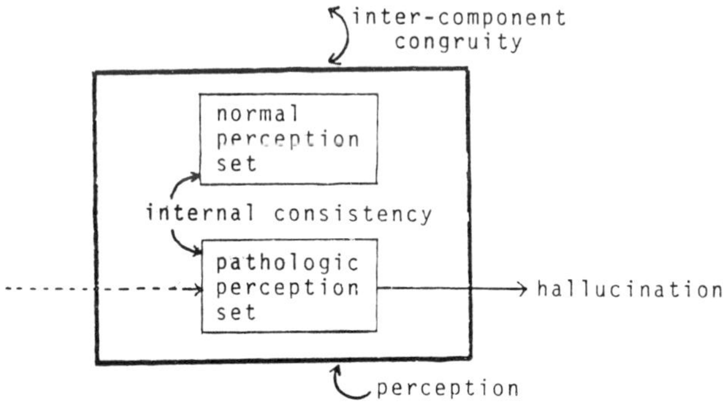

Figure 6

tory hallucinations. If visual hallucinations occur exclusively or dominate the mental state, they suggest that the psychosis is of organic etiology. No hallucination type is pathognomonic for organic versus functional impairment.

At first sight, the schizophrenic may seem to have an alteration in the level of consciousness. This is not a primary delerium of the type seen in acute organic brain syndromes but is a reflection of the incorporated pathological perceptions and thought disorder if one is present. Primary disorientation is not part of schizophrenia. One must get the patient's attention and ask the correct questions. For example, the patient may have a delusion which refers to time having stopped but may respond correctly if asked what time we "incorrectly" think it to be.

The extent of the hallucinations in the schizophrenic's overall perception varies. In general, they do not prevent a clinical interview or totally paralyse the schizophrenic's functioning. In states of *hallucinosis*, they do become so profound and persistent that they dominate the mental state but this is more often an organic psychosis than schizophrenia.

A clinical example is the alcoholic hallucinosis sometimes seen in the withdrawal phase of prolonged alcoholism. The syndrome has two major features similar to schizophrenia. It occurs without a primary alteration in the level of consciousness and the dominant form of hallucinations is auditory. It is important to differentiate alcoholic hallucinosis from delirium tremens. In the latter, there is a primary alteration in the level of consciousness and the hallucinations are generally visual. After recovery from hallucinosis, the patient recalls the hallucinations in detail but in delirium tremens the recall is limited because of the altered level of consciousness.

The auditory hallucinations in schizophrenia, particularly in the early stages of the disease, may be unclear and described as "noises or muffled words." The detail and structure of schizophrenic auditory hallucinations, even in the established case, tend to be limited. Specific content such as

"Hey, let's get together and beat the hell out of the son of a bitch until he is close to dead" is more likely to be reported in a toxic hallucinosis than schizophrenia. The typical content of schizophrenic hallucinations will be discussed later in the section on diagnostic considerations.

Since the hallucinations are "real" from the patient's viewpoint they are processed in a congruent manner by other components of the mental state. A threatening persecutory content will result in an appropriate cognitive, affective and behavioural response. He says, "Of course they scare me, they would scare you too, after all I am not an idiot."

The schizophrenic process may result in a "crossed modality" of perception. Sunlight reflecting off a building is perceived not as different colours or intensities but possibly as pressures, smells or tastes. The patient may report *cenesthesic hallucinations* which involve sensing the functioning of an organ system which has no such perceptive modalities. He may feel the kidney squeezing urine into the ureter or feel thoughts moving across his brain when thinking.

The *somatic hallucinations* are an example of the interaction between psychopathology from different components of the mental state. If the schizophrenic has a persecutory delusion that the Communists are beaming deadly radiation into his house, he reports feeling the effects on his skin. There may be a cenesthesic quality in that they may be perceived in an organ system which in fact has no such modality. Reports of pain deep in the tissue of the cerebral hemispheres would be an example.

It should be mentioned that there is a set of hallucinations not related to an underlying psychotic disorder. Some clinicians refer to these as *pseudohallucinations* but this is troublesome since it suggests that they are false. A better term would be *benign hallucinations*. A single psychotic symptom does not mean a psychosis any more than the single symptom of pain in the left arm means a myocardial infarction. The common benign hallucinations are called *hypnogogic* and *hypnopompic*. The first occur in the drowsy state just before sleep and the latter occur on arousal. Both states occur in a non-pathological altered state of consciousness. Often, the patients are clearly under stress, such as mourning the death of a spouse or some other anxiety-provoking or depression-associated situation.

The hallucination may consist of hearing or seeing a person known to be dead. These are common and normal phenomena under such stressful circumstances. Pointing this out to the person is probably the best form of treatment.

In schizophrenia, the perturbation of perception can result in *illusions*, which are a misperception of a stimulus. As with hallucinations, the primary pathology lies in the perceptual component and the illusion is not rejected as invalid by the normal perceptual sets. An example of an illusion is that a walking stick is processed by a pathological perceptual set and registered in the mind as a sword and is processed as such by the rest of the mental components. This is shown schematically in the following figure.

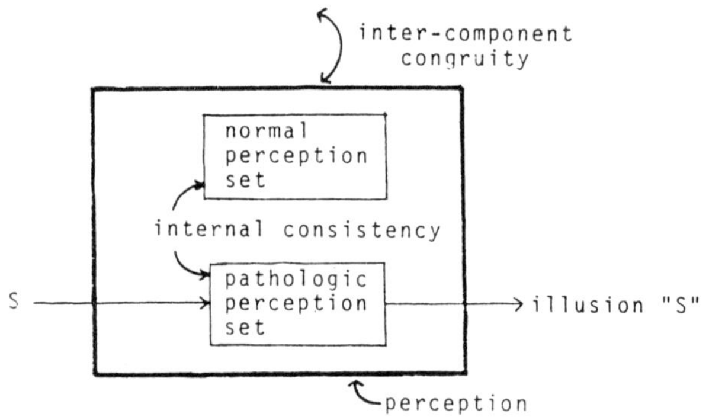

Figure 7

Illusional distortions are not limited to psychotic states. After a few straight days on call in the hospital, a physician may "hear" his name being called when in fact there are only the noises of a busy street. There is no question that for a moment this event is "real" in the mind of the individual. When this perception is reviewed in the context of all the other processes of the non-psychotic mind, it is quickly rejected as a distortion due to being "bushed."

Since the principal components of the mental state are continuously influencing each other, it is sometimes difficult to decide which component is the source of the primary perturbation. This can be illustrated with the aid of the following figure.

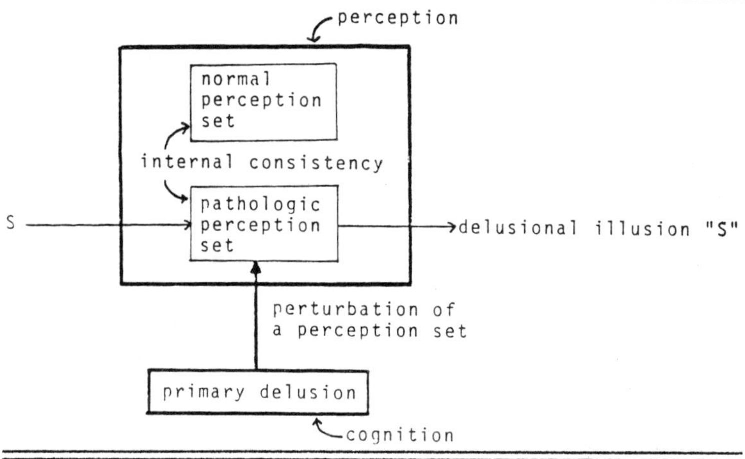

Figure 8

On the one hand, the walking-stick perceived as a sword may be due to a core disturbance in perception and is an illusion. Suppose instead that the core perturbation is in the cognition in the form of a persecutory delusion. This perturbation may spread within the mental state to involve perception and give rise to the same symptoms but now it is a *delusional illusion.*

The difference is not just a matter of "semantics." If the core perturbation was in the affect component, one could develop similar symptoms as described above via extension into the perception and cognition components. The functional psychosis in this case is an affective disorder rather than schizophrenia. The differentiation between the two is crucial since the pharmacotherapy is oriented to *neuroleptics* in schizophrenia and to *thymoleptics* in affective disorders, and are fundamentally different medications.

THE PSYCHOPATHOLOGY OF AFFECT

> Affect refers to a subjective and momentary emotional complex which often has physiological accompaniments. Mood is a feeling state which involves more prolonged and pervasive emotion.

In the schizophrenias, by definition, the psychopathology is not the result of a primary perturbation located in the affect component of the mental state. However, the affect in schizophrenia can be and usually is perturbed. There can be a wide range of affective symptoms including anxiety, anger, fear, depression, elation or loss of affect.

In the early acute phase of schizophrenia, the affect is frequently anxiety. This stage of the developing disease process has been called the *trema phase* which approximately translates as "stage-fright." The patient is aware of alteration in the mental state but no demonstrable overt psychotic symptoms have occured. He says "I have this uncomfortable feeling that something is happening but I am not sure what, why or how."

Such "free floating" anxiety or non-ascribable feelings of apprehension, tension, dread and uncomfortableness are associated with physiological accompaniments such as tachycardia, tachypnea, dizziness and dry mouth. It is a painful situation.

The anxiety level of the trema phase may escalate to the point of a *panic attack* and the patient begins to "lose executive control" of his functioning. Finally, the psychotic symptoms such as a delusional perception or a frank hallucination become manifest. Ironically, this is often a relief for the patient since "Now I know what is happening and can at least face the situation."

Once the schizophrenic disorder becomes entrenched in the mental state, the schizophrenic process has perturbed many, if not all, components to some degree. The affect is congruent with many of the mental processes. This will be true for both the pathological and non-pathological mental sets.

Delusion of persecution may elicit a range of *congruent affect responses* such as fear, anger and hostility. A gradiose delusion may result in an affect that is elated or serene. Similar congruent responses may be seen to other psychotic symptoms such as hallucinations. In addition, the schizophrenic continues to respond congruently to life's stresses as do others unless these stresses have been incorporated into the psychotic symptoms. He may enjoy parties, grieve at funerals, be upset by insults and worry about family problems. His affect continues to be modulated, responsive and expressive despite the invasion of the schizophrenic process into the mental state. It should be stressed that schizophrenia rarely, if indeed ever, totally "paralyses" the mental functioning of the patient.

It should be noted that schizophrenics are subject to all the other medical problems seen in non-psychotics. The schizophrenic is not oblivious to the pain and difficulties associated with other disorders. It is pathetic to see a patient inappropriately not treated and "turfed" without adequate consideration of such problems because the patient has a past psychiatric diagnosis. This situation occurs at an alarming rate.

In the latter stages of schizophrenia, or earlier if the process is particularly malignant, a *fragmentation* occurs within the mental state. The components of the mental state no longer act in concert but display features of *incongruity*. This is most readily apparent in the affective responses. The patient may report a persecutory delusion but the accompanying affect is one of *indifference* and *blandness* rather than the earlier fear, anger or hostility. In fact, the patient may cognitively reason that his mood should be one of fear or anger but experience no emotion or only one which is *blunt, flat* and *poverty-stricken.*

An individual's *personality* consists of a set of habitual responses. Factors involved in responses include the existing mental set, external events, and, most importantly, a vast array of habit patterns formed to deal with developmental influences over his whole life-span. Many of these critical habit patterns are developed in childhood and modified during adolescence. A person's set of emotional responses is one of the main items used to summarise his personality. For example, one is described as the sort of person "who easily loses his temper" or as a "sad and depressed character."

Incongruities between the mental state components by fragmentation can become a characteristic in the schizophrenic, Often, a change in personality is the first indication of the invasion of the mental state by the schizophrenic process. Since affect is a primary characteristic in the ascribing of the personality, its fragmentation and incongruity are often quickly noticed.

A frequently used term in discussion of schizophrenia is the *splitting of the personality.* This does not refer to the creation of multiple personalities but rather the fragmentation of the single pre-morbid personality of the patient. The incongruities and loss of functioning in concert of the components result in the "splitting off" of many of the patient's normal characteristics.

Classically, the severe and chronic schizophrenic process results in a lack of affect response which is described as flat or blunted. The patient is frequently described as a "shell of his former self." An elderly schizophrenic can easily be misdiagnosed as having dementia or an organic brain syndrome. This is unfortunate since treatment would improve the patient's lot in life. It should be noted that this poverty of affect could be a symptom of an affective disorder rather than schizophrenia.

Often, the word *inappropriate* is used instead of incongruent. This can be misleading and can be a sociological judgment. It may be inappropriate for the schizophrenic to be standing on a street corner giggling to himself. However, this affective response may be congruent to an hallucination or delusion of which the observer is unaware. If so, fragmentation of the mental state is not as severe as the observation would suggest. It is "inappropriate" for an adolescent to smile upon hearing of his father's death but the smile and callous comment may be immature defenses to avoid breaking into tears. Similar "gallows humor" is common in intensive care units and terminal oncology wards.

Affective responses are cardinal factors in a person's ability to develop and maintain interpersonal relationships. A cold and unmodulated affective response and, even more so, one which is incongruent, leads to social isolation. The symptoms of the patient accelerate the overall deterioration as the primary psychopathology adds secondary social pathology. Patients get the reputation of being "weird," or "freaky" and are soon shunned by others.

THE PSYCHOPATHOLOGY OF MOBILITY

> Mobility refers to the mental representation of will, drive and volition which initiates voluntary speech and movement.

The act of scratching one's nose is magnificant in its complexity. The neuronal tracts, the brain structures and the muscle groups interact with amazing synchrony. The origin of the act can be ascribed to neuronal receptors in the brain cortex but no matter how reductionistic the model there is the problem of the *mind-body* or *psyche-soma* interface.

There remains the question, "What kicks off the receptor?" and, "What kicks off the unit that kicks off the receptor?" One is forced to invoke *volition* as a mental set comprising "the will to," "the drive to" or the "urge to" as the mechanism to turn on the organic system.

It is remarkable how conveniently a clinical problem can be ignored or minimised by saying that "It is all in the mind."

Ironically, this is mostly done whilst denying the mind actual validity.

The corresponding clinical attitude is to say that the symptoms of a patient with "a normal total body scan" are "all in his mind." This implies that the symptoms are not "real." Renal colic is "real" pain if the stone is demonstrable on x-ray but not otherwise? The arrogance is both outrageous and pathetic.

The symptoms which arise from a perturbation of the mobility component of the mental state are seen in the clinical syndrome of *catatonia*. The syndrome of catatonia has a range of possible organic as well as functional etiologies. *Catatonic schizophrenia* is one of the latter. The catatonic symptoms characteristically manifest as motor or speech abnormalities which can be viewed as features of verbal and non-verbal language.

The symptoms reflect a primary perturbation of mobility and its extension into cognition, perception, affect or behaviour. *Mannerisms* are personalized verbal or motor gestures. An individual may say "God damn it" whenever needing to stress a point, another may draw deeply on a pipe when pondering an important response. In the majority of cases, mannerisms are neither morbid nor pathological but simply reflections of the personality.

Tics are more pronounced and more likely to be pathological. The classic example of severe tics is in the syndrome of Gilles de la Tourette. Here, a young patient presents with facial twitching which progessively increases in frequency and complexity. Later, these motor tics are joined by verbal tics, the latter initially uncontrollable grunting which may develop over time into uncontrollable profane utterances or *coprolalia*. The current evidence is that this syndrome is of organic etiology involving aspects of the limbic system.

In schizophrenia, the agitated catatonic symptoms may present as *stereotypies*. The motor stereotypies may consist of the schizophrenic performing "jumping jacks" or "twirling" continuously for hours with amazing stamina. The patient may explain that the mobility symptoms were in response to auditory hallucinations or were based on a delusional conviction that unless they continued he or someone else would die.

The schizophrenic verbal stereotypies may be the repeating of a phrase such as "that is for me to know and you to find out." Again, this could be a congruent response to a repeated auditory hallucination or based on a formal thought disorder which sees the clinician's questions as dangerous or threatening.

The verbal stereotypie may have a *stilted* quality, for example, "We are pleased to receive that utterance from your personage." If this is given in response to every question, it may serve as a means to maintain the schizophrenic's isolation from what he pathologically assesses to be a dangerous assault.

Echopraxia is a motor symptom reflecting a mobility problem in which the schizophrenic mimics the actions of the examiner. The verbal equivalent is *echolalia* where the patient repeats the words said to him. These behaviours maintain the protective isolation of the patient and may be a reflection of the patient's *poverty of ideation.*

The above examples were discussed in terms of mobility pathology being an extension of a perturbation of other components of the mental state. A primary disturbance of mobility resulting in a distortion of volition may be implied by features of *passivity*. Here, the schizophrenic's mental state is beginning to lose the fundamental feature of *autonomy.* The patient's thoughts and actions show signs of being impelled, controlled, and *made to* to the point of his becoming an *automaton*. This is part of the personality fragmentation leading to a loss of the *integrity of the self.*

There is a range of severity of the symptoms in agitated catatonic schizophrenia up to the point of a bizarre and hyperactive rage. The symptoms are an indication of the pathological sets which exist in the patient's mental state.

The commonest catatonic schizophrenia is the retarded rather than the agitated type. There is a similar wide range of severity in the verbal and motor symptoms. In the extreme case, the schizophrenic is mute and comatose. The differential diagnosis of possible organic etiologies is extensive as was the case in the agitated type. It must be noted that even if this is found to be a functional problem, the patient is in danger from a number of sequelae such as fluid and electrolyte imbalance and pneumonia. Also, if the problem is of functional etiology, it could represent an affective disorder displaying marked psychomotor retardation rather than schizophrenia.

A characteristic of hypomobility in schizophrenia is *flexabilitis cerea* or waxy flexibility. The limbs display a sustained "waxy" dystonia as they are positioned by the examiner. When released, the limb remains in that position for several minutes even if it is uncomfortable and distorted. The limb may remain as placed for a prolonged period of time before slowly "melting" back to a normal resting position. An example is the "psychic pillow" in which the schizophrenic lies motionless on the bed with his head held some six inches above the mattress for a prolonged period of time.

Flexabilitis cerea should be differentiated from *catalepsy*, which is found in states of hypnosis or dissociate hysteria. In catalepsy, the limb offers no resistance to being positioned by the examiner and upon release remains only after an increase in muscle tone or else flops down onto the bed often in a "dramatic" fashion.

As with the symptoms of agitated catatonic schizophrenia, the symptoms of retarded catatonic schizophrenia may be a congruent response to hallucinations or delusional ideation or may represent passivity of volition. The term stereotypies is applicable to both the agitated and retarded symptoms with the former being a "positive" phenomenon and the latter a "negative" phenomenon.

The similarities between the symptoms seen in disorders of mobility and organic problems involving the basal ganglia are noteworthy. Both problems involve a dystonia which in one case is called "waxy" and in the latter, "lead pipe" limb.

The functional and organic syndromes both display a dyskinesia. There are repetative verbal and motor rituals in the functional and choreoathetosis and tremors in the organic problem. Both symdromes can display negative phenomena such as posturing and varying degrees of akinesia. These common features reminds one of the psyche-soma interface.

THE PSYCHOPATHOLOGY OF BEHAVIOUR

Behaviour is defined as all those observable actions which establish and influence interpersonal relationships and have a major influence on the lifestyle.

Given the nature of the symptoms in schizophrenia and the manner in which they are integrated into the mental state, it is obvious that behaviour will be affected. It is possible that the symptoms are such that others remain unaware of change in behaviour. It may be upsetting to many people that schizophrenics are not automatically identifiable.

Subtle changes in behaviour are frequently the earliest indication of the disorder but are often only apparent in retrospect. This is an important piece of information to be considered in the making of a diagnosis. A change in personality or behaviour such as the "straight A's" student becoming withdrawn and morose should not be taken in isolation as indicating schizophrenia. However, such a change in association with other symptoms is a common feature of the onset of schizophrenia.

Classically, the schizophrenic, perhaps initially as a congruent response to his psychopathology, will *drift* down the social scale. He enters into a vicious circle which is difficult to interrupt. As a means of coping with the mental pathology and the secondary social problems, the schizophrenic may turn to street drugs or alcohol. Later, it is difficult to separate the "chicken from the egg." It is important in terms of treatment and prognosis to determine whether the personality deterioration or the substance abuse came first.

Classically, the schizophrenic *migrates* to the lower socioeconomic areas of the cities. On the one hand, this may be the simple economics of functioning in an impaired mental state, but on the other hand, it may be easier to cope in a setting of social isolation, given the primary symptomatology. No matter the reasons, once the patient is recognisable as different by his behavior the isolation and downhill course can be rapid.

There is a "defect" state associated with schizophrenia. It is a result of the deterioration in the mental state coupled with the social sequelae. The danger lies in taking the defect state to be totally related to the mental component and considering it to be irreversible.

Even if the patient is correctly diagnosed, medical and social services are in many cases sadly lacking. Frequently, despite their availability, they are not accepted by the patient. There is a likelihood that the patient enters a "revolving door" between the street and poor treatment facilities.

When successfully treated, he had best not admit to having had schizophrenia because of the stigma and prejudice associated with the disorder. This situation does little to help remove the incorrect notions ascribed to schizophrenia.

Schizophrenia is not a "meaningful voyage of self discovery" as some would argue. Anyone who has dealt with a psychotic patient and his distraught family in the emergency room is aware of the utter ridiculousness of that viewpoint. The approach of "Well, Mr. Bruno, I suggest that you take Stanley home and when this has resolved you will all see that this has been a splended exercise in self awareness" is not helpful. This disorder is neither a "myth" or a "means of political oppression." The point is quickly brought home when the person in the cubicle is a colleague or relative who cannot be simply "turfed" as a "wierdo."

CHAPTER 3

DIAGNOSTIC CONSIDERATIONS IN THE SCHIZOPHRENIAS

For all clinical problems, the diagnostic considerations are a reflection of the *zeitgeist*. They are a reflection of the total body of medical knowledge and opinion available at that point in time. The "Great Pox" of the Middle Ages was a forerunner of syphilis but probably included under its heading other disorders which today can be differentiated from syphilis. Similarly, "madness," as described throughout medical history, includes today's schizophrenias, affective disorders and a range of mental disturbances of organic etiology.

At the outset, diagnostic considerations are of necessity broad and overinclusive. They begin to resolve into subgroups as medical knowledge increases. This differentiating knowledge results from deliberate and accidental observations of the natural course and outcome, signs and symptom clustering, genetic and familial information, treatment methods and responses and laboratory data of the disease. An ongoing reassessment of this data is necessary to prevent bias and error.

At the center of the diagnostic consideration is the differential diagnosis. This takes into account both the pros and cons of each item in order to focus on the most likely diagnosis. This approach is crucial, given the lack of pathognomonic factors in clinical disorders. A high blood glucose is not pathognomonic of diabetes mellitus nor is a positive rheumatoid factor diagnostic of rheumatoid arthritis. Such single items must be considered in a total review of the clinical presentation. The presence of hallucinations or delusions are not exclusive to the functional psychoses let alone to schizophrenia.

The following discussion of diagnostic features of the schizophrenias reflects the zeitgeist as order is brought to the spectrum of functional pyschoses and the group referred to as the schizophrenias. As one reviews the earlier diagnostic considerations, their biases, as imposed by the investigational instruments available at that time, are apparent. Despite the limitations the information is very valuable in developing an understanding of the schizophrenias.

KRAEPELIN

In the nineteenth century, few psychoses were of demonstrable etiology. The model for psychotic disorders was central nervous system syphilis in the form of General Paresis of the Insane (GPI). Treatment of the psychotic disorders was custodial and palliative with discussion about the value of humane versus restraint-oriented care. Classification focused on the natural course of the disorders.

Kraepelin described with great skill the psychopathology of his psychiatric patients and paid particular attention to their clinical course. This led him to divide the psychoses into two major groups. For this he and the German school of medicine must be credited with bringing order to the general concept of psychoses. The two groups were the *manic-depressive disorders* and *dementia praecox*. The latter, dementia praecox, is the forerunner of the schizophrenias.

Dementia praecox was noted to begin insidiously in adolescence, this early onset resulting in the word praecox. The natural course of the disorder was one of steady deterioration in mental functioning resulting in an end state similar to dementia of organic etiology. Once this downhill course started, there was no return to the premorbid level of functioning and usually no arrest period in the deterioration. The diagnosis of dementia praecox implied a fatalistic view.

These characteristics now appear to be a gross oversimplification but given the zeitgeist at the time, this was understandably necessary. Probably, a number of present day organic disorders were unrecognised and included under the heading of dementia praecox. Given the general hospital facilities for many patients at this time and the outpatient services, continued downhill course may have reflected secondary social problems to some extent.

The clinical course of dementia praecox was in marked contrast to that of manic-depressive disorders. The latter had a series of relapses and remissions. During the remissions, the patient returned to the level of premorbid function. The manic-depressive patients tended to have onset in their twenties rather than in adolescence as was prominent with dementia praecox.

Using the dominant psychopathology, Kraeplin divided dementia praecox into three components. These were *dementia praecox paranoides, dementia praecox hebephrenic* and *dementia praecox catatonic.* The dominant symptom in the first subgroup is a delusion; in the second, a thought disorder; in the third, a disturbance of mobility.

```
                  ┌-dementia praecox paranoides (delusion)
dementia praecox ─┼-dementia praecox hebephrenic (thought disorder)
                  └-dementia praecox catatonic (mobility)
```

Figure 9

Follow-up studies of dementia praecox patients showed that deterioration to end stage "dementia" was not inevitable. This led some critics to suggest these cases be called dementia praecox without dementia. The finding simply illustrated that dementia praecox was no different from other clinical disorders in having a range of severity.

All the varieties were observed to be recurrent and for the most part to be associated with increasing severity with a lack of return to the premorbid baseline personality. In these respects, dementia praecox was more "malignant" than the affective disorder of manic-depressive illness.

BLEULER

In the early part of this century, Bleuler reviewed dementia praecox with an alternative diagnosis of *the group of schizophrenias*. He stressed that rather than a single entity, they were a group of disorders. Bleuler pointed out that the loss of mental functioning was not a permanent loss as with organic dementia but a "splitting off" of access to certain normal mental functions which could and occasionally did return.

He pointed out that, as with all clinical disorders, the course and outcome were variable and depended on the severity of the disorder in the given patient. This is illustrated in the following figure.

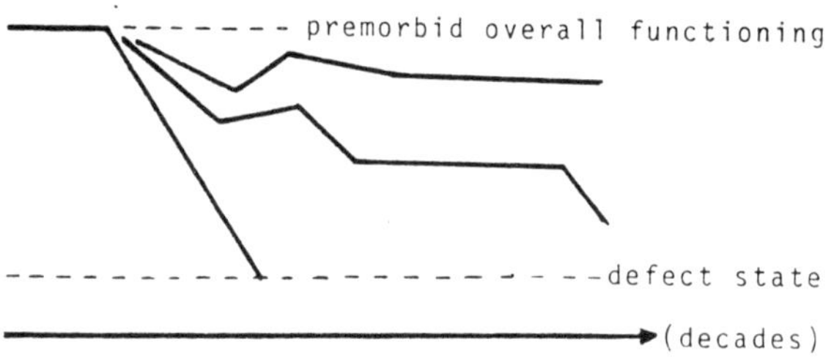

Figure 10

Some cases showed a relentless deterioration akin to Kraepelin's dementia praecox whereas others had an intermittent course with significant periods of arrest in the deterioration and some had degrees of partial improvement. It is possible that a complete arrest without further deterioration could occur before the "dementia" end state was reached. No matter the type of course followed in schizophrenia, the full premorbid functioning was never reattained. There was no "restitutio ad integrum."

The psychoanalytic theories of Freud and his followers were of some interest and Bleuler used some of the concepts in his diagnostic considerations of the schizophrenias. He stressed the fundamental defects of the schizophrenic process which became known as *Bleuler's 4a's*. These are commonly given as *associations, affect, autism* and *ambivalence*. The frequently omitted fifth "a" is *absence* which refers to such a disturbance of memory suggesting an organic-like deficit.

The fundamental symptoms of schizophrenia relating to disturbance of associations have been discussed earlier in this text as were the symptoms arising from a perturbation of affect.

In order to discuss autism and ambivalence, it is necessary to briefly outline some psychoanalytic concepts. A central feature of the Freudian model is that the presence of psychotic symptoms suggests a *regression* has taken place in the mental functioning. That is to say, there has been a re-emergence of mental processes which normally are present only in the first year or so of life into the mature mental state. The re-emergence of these *primitive processes* influences cognition, perception, affect, mobility and behaviour. The term regression is frequently used in a less intrapsychic sense. The geriatric or post-head trauma patient who now babbles rather than talks or has the bladder control of a six month old child is said by some to be regressed.

In the normal progressive development of mental functioning, the *autistic phase* comprises the first six months of life as described by Freud. During this segment of normal maturation, the mental processes are at their most primitive. As yet, there are no cognitive sets capable of logical reasoning or perceptual sets registering adult-like exteroceptions. At the same time, the affect, mobility and behavioural components of the mental state are rudimentary.

One crucial concept not developed during the autistic phase is the *concept of self*. There is no notion of the uniqueness and integrity of the personality. Independence of functioning of the personal self is not realised. Since there is no concept of self, there is no corresponding *concept of non-self*.

Some symptoms in schizophrenia reflect a regression to similar primitive mental functioning. Some can be grouped in the Bleuler diagnostic consideration under the heading of autism. Symptoms indicating distortion of self and autistic functioning include passivity of volition, ideas of reference, hallucinations and catatonia. These features will be described in detail in the next set of diagnostic considerations of Schneider.

Towards the end of the normal autistic phase, more mature mental sets develop which include concepts of self and non-self and as a result there is a rudimentary notion of *object-relations*. The object relations in a mental state involve more than visual-spatial properties, object-relations include affective and cognitive sets which become integrated with the perceptual set. Most individuals have roughly similar perceptual sets of the President but notably different object-relations. This is because of quite individual affective and cognitive sets influenced by equally individual value systems.

In the mature adult mental state an object-relation is a single composite with "good" and "bad" portions within a single representation. In the primitive form, characteristic of the early stages of mental maturation, an object-relation is not merged into a single composite unit. In the rudimentary form, the "good" and "bad" portions coexist as a pair of equal though antithetical representations. These "opposites" are not considered inconsistent and contradictory by the primitive mental state. This is similar to loosening of associations allowing pathological and non-pathological mental sets to "peacefully" coexist in the schizophrenic mental state.

The re-emergence in object-relations of coexisting but antithetical representations is indicative of regression and the resulting symptoms are grouped in the Bleuler diagnostic consideration under the heading of *ambivalence.*

The term ambivalence as used in general conversation implies that a person has difficulty making up his mind or is aware of mixed features. For example, "I am not sure how I feel about my wife; on the one hand, there are some good things about her but on the other hand, there are things which are bad." This is not ambivalence in the Bleulerian sense associated with schizophrenia. The object-relationship to the wife is a single composite representation with good and bad parts.

In the regressed schizophrenic, the wife is dually represented by a "good" and a "bad" set within the mental state. Pathological ambivalence is not a question of "weighing up the pros and cons." It is a "psychotic indecisiveness" which is not resolved because the need for a unitary resultant opinion is not recognised. In schizophrenia, this ambivalence can present as problems with cognition, affect, perception, mobility and behaviour which can, in the extreme, paralyze mental functioning.

Using the 4a's as a diagnostic framework to group the symptoms seen in the schizophrenias, Bleuler proposed four subtypes, namely, *paranoid schizophrenia, hebephrenic schizophrenia, catatonic schizophrenia* and *simple schizophrenia.* The first three were named for their dominant psychopathology in the same manner used by Kraepelin. The first has a delusion as its dominant symptom; the second, a thought disorder; and the third, a disorder of mobility.

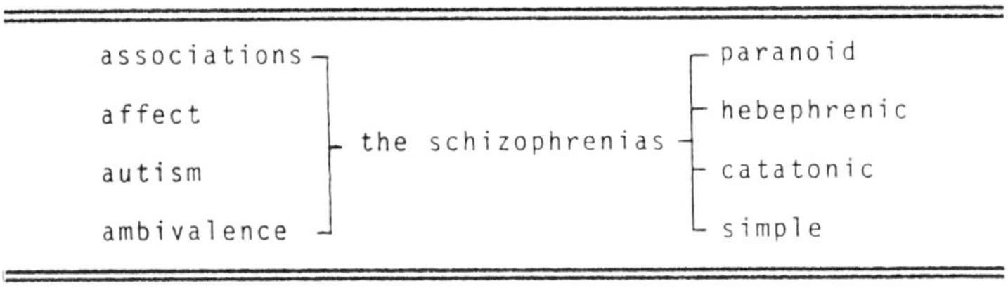

Figure 11

The fourth subtype, simple schizophrenia, has as its dominant symptom a distortion or generally a loss of affect. The central perturbation is not located in the affective component as in the case of the affective disorders, but rather the schizophrenic process manifests itself in this component.

An interesting and informative view of the symptoms of schizophrenia comes from a "need versus fear" model outlined by Bleuler and Freud. As regression takes place involving a part of the mental state, the immediate result may be one of "fear." This relates to the trema phase discussed earlier in reference to the acute schizophrenic breakdown. In order for the mental state to "cope," with this *intrapsychic conflict* and restore *intrapsychic equilibrium* the patient may "need" to create mental symptoms.

As an illustration, the trema phase anxiety expressed as "I have this uncomfortable feeling that something is happening but I am not sure what, why or how" may have the "fear" eased by the development of a delusional perception or hallucination. The symptoms serve a "need" but are pathologically derived in the face of the intrapsychic turmoil.

Another example of the "need versus fear" model in psychoanalytic theory is the possible origin of paranoid ideation. The intrapsychic turmoil produced by a range of intrapsychic conflicts can be eliminated and equilibrium restored by the *externalisation* of the conflict using the *unconscious mental defense mechanism of projection.* A simple example of projection is the senile patient who misplaces items as a result of failing memory, and as a means of coping with this anxiety provoking situation concludes that people are robbing him. Acceptance of the memory loss is neither recognised nor required.

SCHNEIDER

This set of diagnostic considerations moves away from the interperative and psychodynamic approach to one that is more phenomenological or descriptive. The symptoms are taken directly as given by the patient and evaluated independently of theories and preconceptions. It is akin to collecting and assessing the symptoms of a myocardial infarction, in that one is concerned about the *actual form* of the symptom rather than its *symbolic content.*

There are many clinicians who feel that attention to the form rather than the symbolic content reduces the biases and makes for a more objective approach to diagnosis. As an illustration, the form of an auditory hallucination may be two voices which comment on the particular patient's behaviour. The content of what is said and its symbolism is unique to the given patient and is a result of his "overall life history." In the phenomenological approach, the symptom of note is that schizophrenics experience commentary auditory hallucinations. The patients having a myocardial infarction report radiating chest pain but the specific description and symbolism is not the issue.

The following six subheadings outline the *first rank symptoms* of the Schneiderian criteria of schizophrenia. It should be stressed that they are frequent in, but not pathognomonic of, schizophrenia. As many as twenty percent of affective psychoses present with one or more of these symptoms. These symptoms are also encountered in organic psychoses.

1. Hallucinations

There is a particular form of *auditory* hallucination occuring in a clear consciousness. The hallucinations are voices discussing the patient, arguing about the patient or commenting on the patient's behaviour. If the patient is referred to in the hallucination, it is characteristically in the third person.

2. *Echo de pensee*

This symptom consists of the patient's hearing his thoughts out loud like an echo. The train of thought is heard in its entiriety after the patient has carried it through. It is possible, though much rarer, for the "echo" effect to precede the train of thought. One patient said, "My thoughts come to me in my ear, do you see what I mean, doctor?" As will be seen in the next subheading, this has features of thought insertion.

3. Formal thought disorder

There are a number of particular forms of thought disorder considered as first rank symptoms. It should be mentined once again that this criteria is concerned with the form of the thought disorder and not what provokes or comprises the train of thought.

A characteristic symptom is that the patient reports his mind suddenly going blank in mid-sentence. This is the rank symptom of *thought blocking*. The patient frequently says it is as if the thoughts are being actively removed from his mind. This is the characteristic *thought extraction* and must be distinguished from the patient's train of thought stopping due to anxiety or embarrassment. Also, it is important to differentiate thought blocking of schizophrenia from similar symptoms in organic brain syndromes or in the depressed phase of the manic-depressive disorder. Here, the problem is a primary loss of memory function for the first and a lack of concentration in the latter which results in losing track of one's thoughts.

The reporting of thoughts which the patient denies are "his own" represents the symptom of *thought insertion*. Again, there is suggestion of external influence and an "alien" quality. The form of the thought disorder has features of passivity and control. The occurrence can result in symptoms given in other diagnostic considerations such as poverty of thought, tangentiality, overinclusivity and derailment.

Thought insertion should be differentiated from ruminations and obsessive thinking seen in obsessive-compulsive neuroses and depressive disorders. In these cases, the patients report persistent intrusion of unwanted thoughts but the thoughts are their own and lack the alien quality associated with the rank symptoms of schizophrenia.

Another first rank form of thought disorder involves the patient's reporting that his thoughts are not contained in his mind. He feels that they diffuse out from his mind during the thinking process. This *thought broadcasting* or *thought diffusion* may be reported as "people can read my mind." It is important to differentiate this from the common feeling that close friends can anticipate one's thoughts in the sense of, "My wife can read my mind: she knows when I want a cup of tea."

Autistic thinking has been outlined with reference to primitive processes, loss of self concept and breakdown of the integrated personality. These first rank symptoms of thought disorder are excellent illustrations of this situation. Maintaining "executive control" over thought at the basic level is a salient feature of the unperturbed mental state. A normal person's thoughts are influenced by other people and external events or experiences but not at the primary level indicated by the Schneiderian first rank symptoms. These symptoms would fall under the heading of autistic thinking in the Bleulerian diagnostic set and suggest features of the Kraepelinian dementia process. Clearly, the different diagnostic considerations overlap and represent different ways to describe the same feature of the functional disorder.

4. Passivity

These symptoms show similarities to the autistic and ambivalent features. The first rank symptoms of *passivity* have implications of control, influence and "made to" which may involve a number of the components of the mental state.

Thought insertion and withdrawal suggest *passivity of cognition*. In the more marked situation, the complaint has gone from "Some thoughts are not mine, it is as though they are being put there" to the patient reporting "My thoughts are being controlled; I do not have any that are mine." From the cognitive point of view, the passivity has resulted in features of an automaton.

Passivity may involve the affect. The patient reports his affect is not "derived and controlled by me." The *passivity of affect* results in the patient's taking on automation-like features for this component of the mental state. The most critical phase is when passivity involves volition. The initiation of mental processes develops a "made to" quality. The *passivity of volition* reduces the patient to being "a puppet on psychic strings." Passivity of volition suggests an extreme breakdown of ego integrity with regression to a primitive autistic phase.

5. Somatic hallucination

This is a pathological introception. The patient may "feel" thoughts being inserted or extracted from his brain or he may perceive sensations on his skin resulting from "radiation being beamed by the Soviets." These particular types of perception are hallucinations because they lack an external stimulus, and, in many cases, a physiological receptor.

6. Delusional perception

The "two memberedness" of perturbed cognition producing delusional perceptions has been discussed in detail earlier in the text. The perception component is normal but it is coincidentally processed by two cognitive sets, one of which is pathological and the other non-pathological.

The stress is on the form of the symptom rather than the content. The content of a primary delusion or delusional perception of a wealthy lawyer will be different than that of a poor migrant worker. However, both experience the same form of symptom and both will respond to the same medication. The content of such symptoms due to an organic psychosis, for example, due to thyrotoxicosis, would be markedly different for these two individuals but both would respond to the same thyroid suppressing agents.

Secondary complications in the two patients described, whether due to functional or organic psychoses, will be different. This is equally true if the problem is a broken leg, rather than a psychosis.

The discrete first rank symptoms described above are frequently merged in the clinical presentation of the patient. A delusional perception can quickly develop as a persecutory delusion referring to the Soviets and killer satellites beaming death rays onto the patient. This may progress to involve passivity of thinking and behaviour, experiencing body sensations and auditory hallucinations.

This blending of the symptoms is more likely if the psychosis has been present for some time. Discrete first rank symptoms indicate a better prognosis with treatment for the current psychotic episode because it implies a disorder early in its course. It does not imply that the long term prognosis for the disorder is more favourable. Passivity of volition is the first rank symptom indicating a more "ominous" short term prognosis.

In more chronic cases, the first rank symptom may not be ellicitable. In such cases the diagnostic criteria outlined by Bleuler may be of more clinical use. This situation is no different from a range of other medical disorders where the presenting symptom complex is a function of duration of the illness.

Affect symptoms stressed in the Bleulerian diagnostic set are not Schneiderian first rank symptoms. Affect is a first rank symptom only with reference to passivity features. Symptoms such as bluntness and incongruities of affect or visual hallucinations are grouped by Schneider as *second rank* symptoms. The first rank are not pathognomonic of schizophrenia and in many cases it is necessary to make the diagnosis on the basis of these second rank symptoms.

FEIGHNER

Sorting through the differential diagnosis of any clinical disorder uses data in addition to classical signs and symptoms. In schizophrenia, the patient's lifestyle is diagnostically important as is the family history and details of drug abuse.

The Feighner diagnostic considerations are operational criteria particularly useful in chronic cases of schizophrenia. They are divided into three subheadings "weighted" in their contribution to diagnosis.

1. Necessary criteria are:
   a) The clinical disorder has been present for at least six months and during this period there has not been a return to the premorbid level of psychosocial functioning.

   b) There is an absence of clinical features which would indicate the diagnosis of an affective disorder such as manic-depressive illness.
2. At least one of the following criteria is present:
   a) The mental status examination demonstrates primary delusions or hallucinations in the absence of features associated with organicity.
   b) Verbal communication is difficult because of a lack of logical organization due to thought disorder.
3. At least three of the following features need to be present for a "definite" diagnosis and two for a "probable" diagnosis of schizophrenia:
   a) Single marital status.
   b) Indications of poor premorbid social integration such as poor educational, occupational and marital status.
   c) Onset of the disorder prior to age forty.
   d) Absence of drug or alcohol abuse for one year prior to the onset of the disorder.

CHAPTER 4

THE SUBTYPES OF SCHIZOPHRENIA

Clearly, there is a range of symptoms associated with schizophrenia. The form and content of the symptom complex is likely to alter during the course of the illness. The symptom profile and its variations over time will differ from patient to patient. The situation can be viewed in terms of the progressive invasion by the schizophrenic process into the components of the mental state.

The presenting symptom may be restricted to one component of the mental state. This could be in the form of a subtle thought disorder which could undergo minimal alteration over an extended period of time. Alternatively, progression to a form such as a word salad could rapidly occur. At some point in the clinical course, other cognitive symptoms could arise as the schizophrenic process "spreads" within the cognitive component. These could be in a form ranging from limited ideas of reference to frank primary delusions.

The schizophrenic process, with varying degrees of rapidity, may extend to involve other components of the mental state. In some cases, congruency exists between the symptoms from each perturbed component whereas in other cases there is indication of the fragmentation of the composite mental state.

Although schizophrenia is not an infective process, it is instructive to consider a "schizococcus" and ascribe to it "penetrance, virulence and malignancy" along with a given patient's "natural susceptibility and resistance" to the disease.

The subtypes of schizophrenia can be classified in terms of dominant mental symptoms. Accompanying symptoms will depend on the duration and course of the illness and the resultant "malignancy" of the schizophrenic process in the given patient.

HEBEPHRENIC (DISORGANIZED SUBTYPE) SCHIZOPHRENIA

The dominant mental symptom in hebephrenic schizophrenia is a formal thought disorder. This symptom may manifest in a number of forms including loosening of associations, tangentiality, derailment, overinclusivity, interpenetration of themes, failure to maintain a cognitive set, thought blocking, thought insertion, thought withdrawal, thought diffusion and passivity of cognition. It can be exemplified by autistic thinking with its primitive processes, peculiarities of logic and loss of communicative value.

In addition to the definitive thought disorder, other symptoms due to perturbation of the cognitive component may or may not be present. These symtoms may include overvalued ideas, ideas of reference, paranoid ideation and primary delusions. If these symptoms are present or develop at some later point in the course of the illness, they do not dominate the mental state to the degree of the formal thought disorder.

Other components of the mental state can be perturbed in hebephrenia indicating a "spread" of the schizophrenic process beyond the cognitive component. Disturbance of perception can present as misinterpretations, illusions and hallucinations. There may also be symptoms due to perturbation of mobility, affect and behaviour.

The possible symptom profile of hebephrenia is schematically shown in the following figure. The changes that can occur over time are represented in terms of the "penetrance, virulence and malignancy" associated with the schizophrenic process.

Classically, attention is paid to the affect in hebephrenic schizophrenia which has been described as facile, silly, giggly

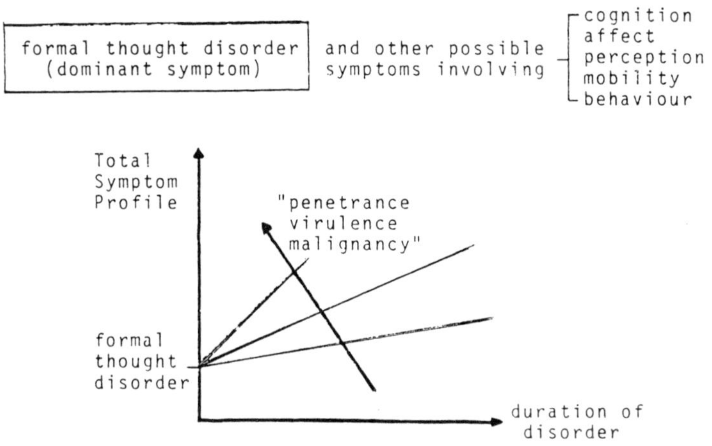

Figure 12

and inappropriate. These features are not due to a primary disorder of affect but are a reflection of the underlying thought disorder. The affect response viewed by an observer as silly and inappropriate may be consistent and congruent with the patient's pathological cognitive processes.

Hebephrenia starts insidiously during adolescence. In the early stages, the first manifestation may be a change or coarsening of the basic personality. The subclinical thought disorder may result in social withdrawal and loss of interest in activities. Only afterwards, when the thought disorder is clinically evident, are these changes recognised as a result of the cognitive perturbation. However, the differential diagnosis of similar changes in personality and behaviour during adolescence includes far more possibilities than early hebephrenia. They may occur in depression, drug abuse and adolescent adjustment reactions.

The disturbance of such a central feature as thought processes in the adolescent period implies a poor prognosis for the development of the individual in many spheres. Limitations and deterioration will be seen in psychological, sociological and educational responses.

CATATONIC SCHIZOPHRENIA

The dominant and definitive symptoms in catatonic schizophrenia arrise from a perturbation of mobility. As discussed earlier, these symptoms cover a spectrum from hypomobility to hypermobility. There is frequently an associated change in verbalisation consistent with the mobility changes.

The most common form of catatonic schizophrenia is the retarded or hypomobile. Classically, there are "poverty" symptoms involving motor behaviour, especially posturing. These unmoving patients are not in coma, although when posturing is coupled with its verbal equivalent of mutism, the presentation is almost identical. These patients are aware of and remember what is being said and done around them.

Often the symptoms can be temporarily reversed by use of intravenous barbiturate or benzodiazepine. This allows some interviewing and aids in diagnosis. This remission of symptoms is shortlived and lasts perhaps ten minutes. It cannot be extended significantly by a steady infusion of the medication over a longer period of time. The classical features of catalepsy and posturing remit when the patients go to sleep.

The differential diagnosis of the retarded catatonic is lengthy. Of the functional etiologies, the catatonic state may be a depressed phase of a manic-depressive disorder with marked psychomotor retardation. Sometimes, during the brief respite with intraveneous barbiturates, information and symptoms can be obtained which substantiate such a diagnosis.

The clinical symptoms may be a conversion reaction or hysterical dissociative response rather than a functional psychosis. This crucial differentiation may be helped by the use of intravenous medication.

The organic etiologies of catatonia are multiple. They range from toxic, metabolic, infectious, and traumatic causes to a variety of conditions involving the central nervous system. Catatonic schizophrenia is one possibility in the differential diagnosis of catatonia, as myocardial infarction is one possibility in the differential diagnosis of chest pain.

There is a great tendency to "blow-off" such patients as hysterics. The workup and management of the retarded catatonic patients bring out the worst in many clinicians. Ironically, they frequently resort to the old cliche "It's all in their head." This can prove embarrassing when the etiology is found to be cerebral oedema due to an undiagnosed brain tumor.

The hypermobile or agitated catatonic schizophrenia is rarer than the retarded form. In general, there is nothing to be gained by using a barbiturate interview. Again, the mobility symptoms dominate the clinical pathology. The verbal equivalents of the hypermobility may be present and demonstrate involvement of other components of the mental state.

In addition to the definitive and dominant mobility symptoms, both the retarded and agitated forms of catatonic schizophrenia can have a range of other symptoms indicating involvement of the other components of the mental state. The interaction of symptoms such as hallucinations and delusions was discussed earlier in the text. The possible symptom profile of catatonic schizophrenia is shown schematically in the following figure.

The symptoms of catatonic schizophrenia are subject to sudden and dramatic changes. The patient who has been in a state of severe retardation may suddenly become hyperagitated. This *raptus* phenomenon makes the catatonic schizophrenic a nursing problem. Sudden eratic behaviour quickly makes the patient a danger to himself and others.

A small number of catatonic schizophrenics have a clinical course with a cyclic nature similar to that seen in the manic-depressive disorders. These infrequent *Periodic Catatonias* were investigated in a systematic manner by Gjessing. He compared their clinical symptoms during relapse and remission phases using a range of biochemical and physiological parameters.

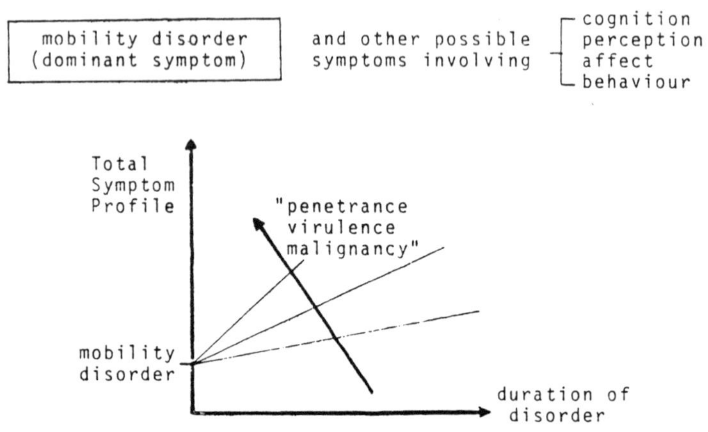

Figure 13

The psychotic relapse phase, whether agitated or retarded in form, varied in duration from patient to patient but for a given patient was relatively consistent and occurred with periodicity. The parameters from either form of psychotic relapse indicated an "adrenergic overactivity." During the interval phase between psychotic episodes, the indication was of "cholinergic excess."

If the psychotic phase, regardless of the form of dysmobility, was related to adrenergic excess a number of medications suggest themselves as possibly useful in treatment. For example, the drug reserpine might alleviate symptoms by promoting release of neurotransmitters from their storage vesicles in the presynaptic terminal. This will allow their degredation by the enzymes located in the presynaptic terminal before they can be released into the synaptic cleft. Disulfram decreases adrenergic neurotransmitters by inhibition of the enzyme dopamine-beta-hydroxylase which is needed for conversion of dopamine to norepinephrine; alpha-methyl-dopa has a similar effect by interference with the enzyme dopa-decarboxylase which normally converts dopa to dopamine. These three drugs had partial but not complete success in the treatment of some patients.

Only one metabolic component, nitrogen balance, correlated with the clinical symptoms of periodic catatonia. This was found to be an endogenous factor unaffected by changes in the patient's diet. Patients found to have a positive nitrogen balance during their remission phase usually had psychotic episodes characterised by retarded catatonia. These patients are designated type A. Patients with a positive nitrogen balance in the psychotic phase, designated type C, invariably had an agitated catatonic phase. A third subgroup of recurrent or periodic catatonia was designated type B. They had positive nitrogen balance both in the remission and psychotic phase and tended to have an agitated catatonic episode. The Gjessing study is an early example of systematic investigation of a functional disorder and illustrates that apparent functional disorders have biological changes if one is sophisticated enough to find them.

Some patients diagnosed as catatonic schizoprenics, because of the clinical symptomatology and lack of demonstrable organic etiology, underwent rapid deteriation ending in death. These patients were variously labelled as *fatal catatonia, lethal catatonia, malignant schizophrenia* and *hypertoxic schizophrenia.* The clinical picture was one of sudden onset of agitated catatonia with rapid deterioration. In addition to the characteristic symptoms of schizophrenia, these patients developed marked hyperthermia. The end stage was death or at best marked neuological deficits upon recovery. Subscquent studies have shown that many of these patients had acute encephalopathies involving the basal ganglia, diencephalon and limbic system. These cases illustrate the "mind-body" interface and the fact that the symptom profiles associated with functional psychoses can be produced essentially "picture perfect" by organic lesions.

Lesions within the central nervous system are often difficult, if not impossible, to identify except at autopsy. Often, such disorders feature alteration in mental function in their clinical presentation. An example of this situation with similarity to catatonic schizophrenia is *akinetic mutism*, or so-called coma vigil. As the name implies, this clinical state is characterised by profound motor and verbal hypomobility. The patients are motionless but their eyes track movement in the room. They cannot chew food but are able to swallow liquids. Suggestive longtract signs such as alteration in pain and proprioception occur along with an alteration in consciousness. These patients may maintain a fetal-like position but are prone to sudden raptus phenomena. The "harried" clinician might write these patients off as a "psych case," particularly if they have a past history of functional disorders. The original case was due to a third ventricular cyst and others have been found with a variety of toxic and organic etiologies.

Of the subtypes of schizophrenia, the catatonic, both retarded and agitated, has the best response to convulsive therapy (ECT). It is the only subtype of schizophrenia for which this treatment is clearly indicated and may, in fact, be the treatment of choice.

Given the rapid improvement after ECT and the fact that the nature of the symptoms lends itself to quick identification and hospitalization, catatonic schizophrenia can be considered as having the best prognosis of the schizophrenias. However, it cannot be overstressed that catatonic symptoms do not necessarily imply catatonic schizophrenia and the differential must be explored.

PARANOID SCHIZOPHRENIA

The dominant and definitive symptom in paranoid schizophrenia is a primary delusion. The commonest delusion is persecutory but paranoid schizophrenia may have grandiose, religious, sexual and somatic delusion content. Taking into account all age groups, paranoid is the commonest subtype of the schizophrenias.

Depending on the duration and "malignancy" of the schizophrenic process, other symptoms may be present in addition to the dominant delusion.

Some paranoid schizophrenics have a "pre-psychotic" personality which can be described as paranoid. In many patients, this paranoid personality represents a significant change from the original personality. In such cases, the new and changed personality could be a manifestation of the schizophrenic process.

Not all paranoid schizophrenics have a preceding paranoid personality that is clearly identifiable as first expression of the schizophrenic illness. Also, not all paranoid personalities go on to develop into paranoid psychoses. There is a demonstrable "linkage" between paranoid personality and paranoid psychosis but it is not an "all or nothing" relationship.

There are three noteworthy paranoid states characterized by a primary delusion. They represent variation in "malignancy" of the schizophrenic process, differing responses to the perturbation of the components of the mental state and deteriorative course of the overall functioning of the patient.

The first of these is *paranoia*. By definition, these patients have an encapsulated primary delusion which does not invade other aspects of mental functioning. The low penetrance of the schizophrenic process leads to little or no deteriation in the mental state even after many years. The components of the mental state maintain congruity and fragmentation of the personality does not occur.

Depending on the content of the primary delusion and the degrees to which it is "walled-off," there will be secondary changes in lifestyle. Regarding psychotic symptoms, it appears that elimination of the primary delusional system would result in a normal mental state. Pure paranoia is rare.

Like paranoia, paranoid schizophrenia has an insidious onset often starting in adolescence. After a number of years, or sooner in more "malignant" cases, it is likely that other psychotic symptoms will have been added to the dominant primary delusion. By age fifty or sixty, it is likely that there is a range of symptoms involving a number of components of the mental state and some indication of personality fragmentation. This is in marked contrast to the paranoia disorder.

Of the subtypes of schizophrenia, the greatest variation in symptom complex, course and possible deterioration is seen in the paranoid schizophrenic. By age fifty or sixty, the schizophrenic process having been present for years, it is likely that incongruencies have occurred. Initially, in the early twenties, the persecutory delusion manifested a congruent affect of fear, anger and hostility but now is one of blandness, apathy and indifference about the persecution.

There is likely to have been systematisation and secondary elaboration of the primary schizophrenic symptoms. These secondary symptoms and features become intertwined with the original presentation producing the wide range of symptom complexes seen with paranoid schizophrenia.

Clearly, the first hospitalization may not coincide with the onset of schizophrenia despite definitive symptoms. Some fifteen percent of women and five percent of men with schizophrenia are hospitalized for the first time in their fifth and sixth decades. These patients constitute the third paranoid state of clinical importance which is called *paraphrenia* or *late paraphrenia.*

In terms of the malignancy and invasion of the schizophrenic process into the mental state, this group lies "between" paranoia and paranoid schizophrenia. This is schematically shown in the following figure.

Paraphrenia has a primary delusion, usually persecutory, as its dominant symptom, but also has other psychotic symptoms such as a formal thought disorder and hallucinations. Fragmentation of the personality is strikingly minimal in these patients. Congruency between the mental state components is maintained. Despite the chronicity of the disorder, for example, the affect related to a persecutory delusions remains that of fear, anger or hostility. Paraphrenics are far from being "burnt-out shells of their former

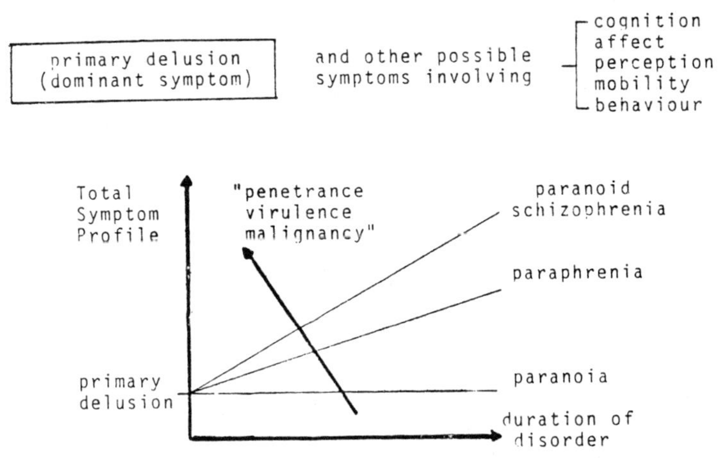

Figure 14

selves" and remain spirited and actively engaged with their psychopathology.

They tend to have had an isolated existence in their neighborhoods for many years and may have been considered "quaint," "touched" and "downright weird" by their neighbors. They may, in their old age, become "regulars" at the police station complaining about problems at the hands of the local mafia or Soviets. It is interesting that as many as forty percent of paraphrenics have problems with deafness which accentuates isolation and paranoid tendencies.

In addition to paraphrenia, such congruent paranoid states in the elderly includes major affective disorders and organic brain symdromes in the differential diagnosis. The differentiation must be done correctly, since the treatment and prognosis for these disorders are very different. The paraphrenics do not show other mental symptoms associated with organic brain symdromes or the rank symptoms of a major affective disorder.

Many paraphrenics are misdiagnosed as organic brain syndromes, particularly if radiological studies indicate cerebral atrophy. At autopsy, the number of plaques seen in paraphrenic brains is less than paranoid states due to organic brain syndromes but more than those seen in similar aged patients with comparable atrophy without mental symptoms.

UNDIFFERENTIATED SCHIZOPHRENIA

In this subtype of schizophrenia, no symptom dominates the mental state. Hence, these cases cannot be assigned to either hebephrenic, catatonic or paranoid schizophrenia. This picture is more likely in chronic cases but lack of a single dominant symptom in the perturbed mental state may occur in the acute phase of schizophrenia.

RESIDUAL (CHRONIC) SCHIZOPHRENIA

One or more episodes of schizophrenia most often results in residual changes in overall function. The psychotic symptoms may persist in a muted form which does not require hospitalization. In other patients, despite treatment, the symptoms may persist to a degree that prevents discharge into the community.

The clinical picture is similar to undifferentiated schizophrenia but previous hospitalizations indicate diagnosis of a paranoid, catatonic or hebephrenic schizophrenia.

In the community, residual schizophrenics can be seen "hanging out." Those circumspect enough to avoid public attention may be the local "bag lady" or "corner preacher." However, it should not be assumed that all such people are schizophrenic. It should also be noted that they are as susceptible to the same illnesses and stresses as other people.

In the state hospitals and nursing homes, many of the long term patients are residual schizophrenics. It is an important question as to whether patients are better off in the understaffed hospital or in a downtown rooming house with little or no attention.

The somewhat irreverent question to be asked is, "Should these burnt outs be put outs?" Many residual schizophrenics illustrate the vicious downward social spiral that results when the mental patient re-enters society. In general, outpatient facilities such as halfway houses and clinics are pathetically inadequate. Much of the patient's problem is social rather than mental.

The preceding five subtypes of schizophrenia are referred to as *process* or *nuclear schizophrenias.* This is because their course and outcome are of the type discussed by Kraepelin and Bleuler as characteristic of dementia praecox and the group of schizophrenias. They constitute the "classical" concept of this functional psychosis.

It is clearly evident in clinical practice that there are a group of functional psychotics who do not follow the classical course. These cases display the characteristic symptoms seen in some schizophrenic patients but differ in a number of significant ways from the classical syndrome. In particular, they differ from the nuclear or process disorder in terms of course and subsequent outcome. Given the variability of the clinical problem it has been stressed that functional psychosis must be viewed on a spectrum. At one extreme, one can speak of classical, nuclear or process schizophrenia whilst at the other pole one can group *non-process* and *non-nuclear* subtypes.

CHAPTER 5

THE ATYPICAL OR NON-PROCESS SCHIZOPHRENIAS

Three clinical subtypes fall under this heading. They are the *schizophreniform*, the *brief reactive* and the *schizo-affective* psychoses.

SCHIZOPHRENIFORM PSYCHOSIS

By definition, the duration of this disorder is longer than two weeks but less than six months. This period must include the prodromal, psychotic and recovery phases. The duration is a principal feature differentiating this atypical form from process schizophrenia.

The onset of schizophreniform psychosis is usually acute and the deterioration to a frank psychotic state is rapid. Generally, the patient or his family can recall a recent point in time when the change in mental functioning occured. Prior to that "Everything was fine. We never dreamed that he would ever need to see a psychiatrist."

The acute onset makes it likely that precipitants will be suggested as "what set the whole thing off." This is in contrast to the patient with process schizophrenia who has an insidious onset. Precipitants should be studied with caution. They may be the result of schizophreniform psychosis rather than the critical factor in onset.

The period of dramatic change in the overall mental function is characterized by stressful events of a psychological and physiological nature. There is a gradual buildup of pressure and a final "straw that breaks the camel's back" is followed by psychosis.

It is not just a specific precipitant but a unique combination of factors coming together at a specific time in the correct proportions to trigger the breakdown. Whether or not this combination is likely to occur again is an important point in the evaluation of the likelihood of recurrence at a later date.

What constitutes stress, varies from person to person and even from time to time in a given individual. In the schizophreniform psychosis, one expects stress factors. A student with numerous problems as he builds up towards a critical examination may fall in this category and an oil-rig worker who has been working around the clock for days under arduous circumstances does so as well. A "flash point" is reached and the psychotic episode is activated.

The content of the schizophreniform psychosis has *understandability*. This does not refer to in-depth comprehension of the symbolism of the symptoms or the unconscious intrapsychic conflicts underlying the psychosis. Understandability implies that what is being communicated by the patient "makes sense," given the apparent stresses, the circumstances, and the nature of the individual. The content of the psychosis is consistent with the time and person involved.

For example, a student talks about academic pressures and personal matters which his family and friends readily identify as being typical for "him." The oil-rig worker's psychotic content is recognized as referring to rigs and personal circumstances. This understandability is in contrast to the classical process schizophrenia where the content is frequently "bizarre" and "not like him at all" from the viewpoint of associates and family.

The atypical schizophrenias have been referred to as *Psychogenic Psychoses*. The content of any psychosis, whether organic, functional of the process or non-process subtype, is a unique product of the patient's own mental state. In the atypical schizophrenias, this psychogenic point is more directly apparent.

Psychotic symptoms in the form of the Schneiderian first rank are likely in the schizophreniform psychosis. This is in keeping with the acute nature of the disorder. The content of these symptoms will have the understandability described but symptoms demonstrating fragmentation of the mental state such as incongruity of affect and content are unlikely.

The schizophreniform psychosis may have periods of altered level of consciousness with episodes of confusion, disorientation and amnesia. These features of alterations in consciousness are not encountered in process schizophrenia. These features of a primary alteration in consciousness force one to consider carefully the possibility of an organic delirium as part of the differential diagnosis. Associates of the patient suggest "He may have been taking street drugs because of the way he was acting." After recovery, the oil-rig worker may not recall the attempt to commandeer the rig's helicopter or the student may not remember pulling the fire-alarms in the dormitory.

The course of schizophreniform psychosis is often characterized by fluctuations in the dominant mental symptoms. This lability is in contrast to the more common constancy of symptoms seen in process schizophrenia. At times, there may be shortlived bursts of manic activity or hysterical symptoms superimposed on the schizophrenic rank symptoms.

The premorbid history of the schizophreniform patient is notable for the lack of features commonly seen in the premorbid schizophrenic. The developmental, social, educational and occupational details are in keeping with the statement that "Everything was fine. We never dreamed that he would ever need to see a psychiatrist." In the same vein, the schizophreniform psychosis patient's family history lacks positive findings relating to schizophrenia.

Frequently asked questions are: Will there be a recurrence of the problem, and will stress increase that possibility? One needs to ask whether a student should return to college or can the oil-rig worker return to the oil fields? The illness can be viewed as a psychosis triggered by a group of particular stress factors coming together at a critical time. The likelihood is that a similar critical cluster of factors will not recur. Therefore, with care in easing the patient back into the premorbid lifestyle, it is likely a recurrence will not take place. It is important to follow the patient closely during his early outpatient phase and address problems that arise within the family and the workplace.

BRIEF REACTIVE PSYCHOSIS

The difference between this atypical psychosis and the schizophreniform disorder is the duration of the brief reactive psychosis, which is by definition less than two weeks. The symptom complex of the two disorders may be identical in the first days of presentation.

Precipitants are more likely to be identified for the brief reactive psychosis than for the schizophreniform disorder. They are more likely to directly trigger the breakdown. It is more necessary to deal with the specific stresses in this case than in the schizophreniform disorder.

The differential diagnosis of the brief reactive psychosis and the schizophreniform psychosis are similar. The adult adjustment reaction is higher on the differential diagnosis list in the brief reactive psychosis than in the case of a process schizophrenia. One should bear in mind the array of toxic-organic conditions which can present in an identical manner as the brief reactive psychosis whether the toxic condition is "street" or "hospital" in origin.

SCHIZO-AFFECTIVE PSYCHOSIS

A dysphoria ranging through anxiety, depression and euphoria can occur in process schizophrenia. Schizo-affective psychosis should not be diagnosed simply because a schizophrenic has dysphoric symptoms. For example, a paranoid schizophrenic who is despondent in response to a persecutory delusion is not schizo-affective.

In the schizo-affective disorder, the affect disturbance is pervasive of the mental state and often is the dominating symptom. Affect symptoms similar to those of the manic-depressive disorders are found but there is fragmentation to a greater extent than is typical in the primary affective disorder of manic-depressive illness. It is as though there is a "mixed" expression of both the schizophrenic and primary affective functional psychoses.

As might be expected, the course and outcome of schizoaffective psychosis is better than for the process schizophrenias. Many feel that this subtype is better classified as an atypical affective disorder than a subtype of schizophrenia.

CHAPTER 6

PERSONALITY DISORDERS ASSOCIATED WITH THE SCHIZOPHRENIAS

Earlier in the text, it was pointed out that change in personality may be indicative of the onset of a schizophrenic process. Given the variability of the pervasiveness of the schizophrenic process and the multitude of factors which define a composite personality, the gradual change in dominant traits of a personality may be the only feature of schizophrenia for a long period of time.

Alterations in character traits need not be related to schizophrenia and such changes need not be progressive or unchangable. Nevertheless, the question arises as to whether there are characteristic premorbid personalities significantly related to schizophrenia. Statistically there is a linkage of certain personality types to schizophrenia but it is far from being an absolute relationship. These personality types may represent, frequently in retrospect, the early or muted expression of the schizophrenic process.

SCHIZOID PERSONALITY DISORDER

Some seventy-five percent of schizophrenics show evidence of an abnormal personality prior to manifesting frank psychotic symptoms. About twenty-five percent have a *schizoid* personality.

A characteristic of the schizoid personality is the inability to form and maintain interpersonal relationships. The first rank symptoms of schizophrenia are absent in a schizoid personality disorder.

The individual is variously described as a loner, shy, withdrawn, isolated and indifferent to interpersonal interactions.

This occurs in adolescent years, which are normally characterized by the development of numerous attachments.

These features are of particular note if they represent a sudden change or arrest in a previously normal personality development. Even when present, there are many possible reasons for such change other than a schizoid disorder, such as a depressive disorder, adolescent adjustment reaction and use of "street" drugs.

It is clear that most persons displaying schizoid features do not go on to later exhibit frank schizophrenia. Also, it is clear that not all schizophrenics show this premorbid personality type in the initial phase of their illness. In view of the stigma associated with the diagnosis of schizophrenia, the term schizoid should not be used indiscriminantly.

PARANOID PERSONALITY DISORDER

The characteristic of this personality is the tendency to employ the unconscious defense mechanism of projection to allay intrapsychic conflict.

The degree of projection is not to the point of producing a delusion and hence a paranoid psychosis. The degree of projection is muted and manifested by suspiciousness, ideas of reference and a tendency ot quickly ascribe one's difficulties to the interference of other people.

Projection becomes a clinical symptom when its employment is of sufficient magnitude to cause problems for the person or others. Not all paranoid personalities necessarily progress to a psychotic state. Once again, there is a statistical relationship to the paranoid schizophrenia but it is not an absolute linkage.

SCHIZOTYPAL PERSONALITY DISORDER

Bleuler, in his discussion of the process schizophrenias, proposed an additional subtype to join the three specified by Kraepelin, namely, *simple* schizophrenia. In the modern classification of the process schizophrenias, it is felt that simple schizophrenia does not warrant a separate subgroup. Simple schizophrenia is now viewed as a personality disorder under the name *schizotypal.*

In the schizotypal individual, the characteristic rank symptoms of schizophrenia are not manifest but the deterioration in mental functioning and accompanying symptomatology is more pronounced than in the schizoid personality disorder. The inadequate interpersonal relationships of the schizoid disorder are seen and they are more disruptive in the schizotypal disorder.

The cognitive component of the mental state reveals impairment of associations, inability to hold a cognitive set and a preoccupation with fantasy and magical thinking but not to the degree of manifesting rank symptoms of schizophrenia. Hallucinations are not present but illusions, misinterpretations, depersonalisation and derealisations occur. Although affective responses may be inappropriate, there are not the incongruities indicative of a fragmentation of the personality associated with process schizophrenia.

Clearly, the behavioural sphere is perturbed in a manner that is morbid for the patient and his associates. The downhill spiral is likely to be evident over a long period of time but the schizophrenic "dementia" is not evident. Ascribing a "malignancy" and "invasiveness" to the pathological process would rate that associated with the schizotypal greater than that of the schizoid but less than that ascribed to atypical or process schizophrenia.

BORDERLINE PERSONALITY

This disorder bears a close resemblance to the older syndrome of *pseudoneurotic schizophrenia.* It is helpful to outline the latter in order to discuss the *borderline* personality.

In pseudoneurotic schizophrenia, frank psychotic episodes with symptoms characteristic of schizophrenia occur sporadically and are sustained only for short periods of time. In atypical schizophrenia, the duration of psychosis is days or weeks but in pseudoneurotic schizophrenia the duration is minutes or a few hours.

These brief psychotic episodes occur against a background of symptoms characteristic of the neuroses. Overall, those symptoms typical of the neuroses dominate the clinical picture. These include anxiety, phobias, obsessive compulsive features and sexual identity problems. These symptoms are poorly delineated and amorphous with fluctuation of the predominant symptom at any given point in time. Thus, the patient is referred to as *pan-anxious* and *pan-neurotic*. During the psychotic period, the patient displays the results of regression but not the *pan-regression* of a florid psychosis.

If the model of an invading schizophrenic process is used, the borderline patient may be taken as a muted expression of schizophrenia which is, however, more "virulent" than that seen in schizoid and schizotypal personality disorders.

The ego functions of the borderline personality are inadequate and often primitive with the ego boundary being tenuously defined. Thus, these patients are relatively poor candidates for conventional psychotherapy. They are notoriously difficult patients to engage in the psychotherapeutic process and termination with lasting positive introjects is not easily achieved. As one would expect, the response to psychopharmacology is limited.

CHAPTER 7

THE ETIOLOGY OF SCHIZOPHRENIA

The first point to be addressed is whether or not a unitary etiology is to be expected for the schizophrenias. The sheer complexity of presentation of this neuropsychiatric disorder suggests that this is unlikely.

There are few, if indeed any, clinical disorders with as absolute an etiology as many students may be lead to believe. Diabetes mellitus is not necessarily due to a "functional insulin deficit." Even when insulin is effectively "low," it is a primary feature but not necessarily the etiology or "cause."

Advances in neurosciences will continue to tease out specific subgroups from the general heading of the schizophrenias. Associated with these advances will no doubt be improvements in the treatment of this clinical syndrome.

Discussing the etiology of the schizophrenias in terms of a "*nature or nurture*" model is pointless and dangerous. From the clinical viewpoint, it is best to leave philosophy to the philosopher but keep some of the points in the back of one's mind. The bias of an "either/or" approach to etiology leads to misdiagnosis and mistreatment. This point is applicable to all medical disorders.

The etiology of schizophrenia is best discussed under three headings: biological, psychological and sociological. They need to be blended together since "man is an act, not a fact."

BIOLOGICAL THEORIES

A discussion of biological etiology should be approached with several questions in mind. Does the biological factor unmask a functional substrate? Does it mimic the disorder when present? Does the biological factor create, de novo, the clinical syndrome? There are organic factors which suggest the first two conditions and perhaps there are indications of the latter.

Head trauma can result in symptoms similar to those seen in schizophrenia. This appears to be more likely if the damage involves the temporal lobe and midbrain regions. The family loading for schizophrenia in these post-traumatic patients is higher than in normal controls but less than that of functional schizophrenics. The suggestion is that the deficits produced by the trauma "releases" a substrate. There is a possibility of the lesions producing the psychotic disorder de novo but this is at most rare and debatable.

The relationship between the epilepsies and schizophrenia is particularly noteworthy. Clinical observations in the 1930's led to the notion of an inverse relationship between epilepsy and schizophrenic symptoms. This led to the use of deliberately induced seizures as a treatment of schizophrenia.

In fact, it appears that there is a higher than expected association of epilepsy and schizophrenia. It has long been observed that symptoms similar to a schizophrenic thought disorder and hallucinations occur in cases of temporal lobe and limbic seizure disorders. This raises the possibility that schizophrenia may be related to dysfunction of the same anatomical areas. It should be noted that temporal lobe or psychomotor seizures may manifest only as a perturbation of the mental state.

Investigation of possible biochemical abnormalities in the schizophrenias is currently focused on the neorutransmitters. For the purpose of this text, the neurotransmitter dopamine will be discussed.

Autopsy of the brains of schizophrenics suggests more dopamine receptors than in the brains of normal controls. Drugs which increase the synthesis of dopamine and/or promote its release into the neuronal synapse can produce organic psychoses which resemble schizophrenia. The drugs which are highly successful in the alleviation of the symptoms of functional schizophrenia block dopamine receptors located on the post-synaptic membrane. This will be discussed in more detail later in the text. The conclusion is that schizophrenia could be related to a perturbation of this neurotransmitter system.

There is a similarity of structure between some of the psychomimetic drugs which produce toxic psychoses similar to schizophrenia and the principal neurotransmitters. Amphetamines promote dopamine synthesis in the brain and can produce a toxic psychosis which very closely mimics schizophrenia. They are structurally similar to dopamine. The psychomimetic psilocybin has a structure similar to the indolamine neurotransmitter serotonin.

Although there is similarity in structure between some of the psychomimetics and neurotransmitters, they differ notably in that the psychomimetics have additional methyl (CH3) groups. The enzyme catechol-o-methyl transferase (COMT) is involved in the normal breakdown of neurotransmitters when it occurs in the synaptic cleft and at the principal site in the pre-synaptic terminal. The *methylation hypothesis* of schizophrenia suggests that this enzyme abnormally methylates, particularly intersynaptically, some normal neurotransmitters in the schizophrenic. If true, this aberrant methylation might result in the schizophrenic manufacturing an "endogenous" psychomimetic. If this and other abnormalities of the neurotransmitter cycle are present, then a small number of these abnormal units might result in a schizophrenic picture.

Support of the methylation hypothesis involves methionine which is a potent donor of methyl groups in neurochemical pathways. Schizophrenics have relapsed into an active psychosis after administration of methionine. These patients had been given a monoamine oxidase inhibitor as well as the methionine since that drug blocks the other enzyme involved in the breakdown of neurotransmitters. Such a combination is felt to amplify the effects of the aberrant methylated units but the technique has a number of epi-phenomena and is imperfect.

The compound MSO is an antimetabolite of methionine. It causes toxic psychoses in normals but not in schizophrenics. The implication is that schizophrenics have effectively higher methionine levels than the controls. In the same vein, there is a suggested higher incidence of schizophrenia in homocystinuric patients than in normal controls. The enzyme deficiency in these patients is cystathione synthetase which converts methionine to other metabolites. The implication is that they have higher methionine levels and would be more prone to aberrant methylation processes.

The *hydroxylation hypothesis* involves the aberrant hydoxylation of the neurotransmitter serotonin (5 hydroxytryptamine). Attempts to identify the aberrant neurotransmitters or their metabolites have been only partially successful. The results of these studies are tantalising but inconclusive.

There have been a number of attempts to identify abnormal biochemical markers for schizophrenia. When the complexity of the neuropsychiatric disorders comprising the schizophrenias is recalled, the likelihood of a consistent marker is placed in perspective. The RF factor is not the marker for arthritis. The latter is a condition whose complexity palls in comparison to the schizophrenias. Potential markers have included such factors as phosphate metabolism, alterations in the immune system, abnormalities in plasma proteins, variations in cellular metabolism and changes in specific enzymes.

It was found that the enzyme CPK was elevated in acute psychoses. This has three principal isoenzymes MM, MB, and BB which derive from skeletal muscle, cardiac muscle and the central nervous system respectively. It is not clear whether the elevation of CPK is a reflection of central nervous system changes during a psychotic episode or of muscle-skeletal and cardiac changes occuring in response to the psychotic state. The problem is complicated because the BB isoenzyme is rapidly converted to an MM fraction.

It is worthwhile expanding on the biological model involving the action of amphetamine. Patients who have abused this drug frequently present in the emergency room, raising the possibility of schizophrenia as a diagnosis. In some cases, the amphetamine psychoses very closely mimic functional schizophrenia. Also, details of the pharmacology of amphetamine is a help in discussing the action of drugs which are effective in treatment of schizophrenia.

Amphetamines flood the dopamine system. They increase activity of tyrosine hydroxylase, which is the rate limiting enzyme of dopamine synthesis. They promote release of dopamine from the pre-synaptic terminal into the synaptic cleft, resulting in increased occupation of dopamine receptors located on the post-synaptic terminal membrane.

The principal site of dopamine breakdown is located in the pre-synaptic terminal and, therefore, dopamine has to undergo an active reuptake across the pre-synaptic membrane for deactivation. This active reuptake is inhibited by amphetamine. The dopamine cycle is schematically shown in the following figure.

The enzymes involved in the breakdown of dopamine in the pre-synaptic terminal include COMT and MAO located in the mitochondria. Amphetamine inhibits the action of these en-

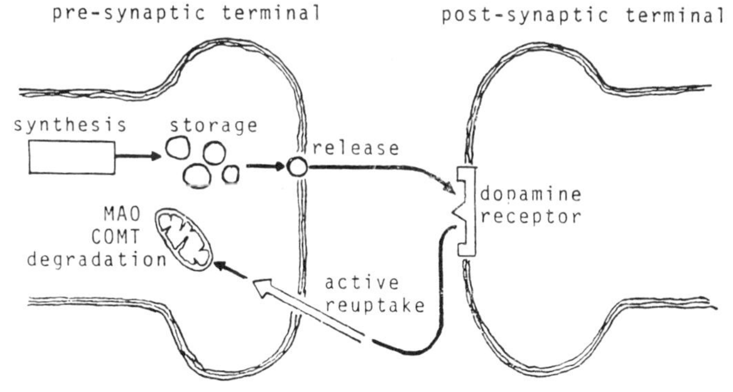

Figure 15

zymes. Therefore, at a number of significant steps, amphetamine "turns on" the dopamine system.

The clinical syndromes produced by amphetamines can be divided into three parts. Firstly, there is a situation due to acute ingestion of amphetamine, either orally or intravenously, which results in a subjective "high." The toxic psychosis can usually be distinguished from functional schizophrenia on a numberof clinical points.

The patient has an alteration in his level of consciusness suggesting an acute organic brain syndrome. Hallucinations tend to be of more than one form, such as visual, somatic and auditory. They are likely to be persistent and intrusive with a detailed content suggestive of hallucinosis. Paranoid ideation is common and tends to be persecutory also it is congruently reflected in labile and impulsive affect and behaviour. The patient tends to be overactive and distractable resulting in serious management difficulties in the emergency room.

A patient with an acute amphetamine toxicity can be described as "freaky" or a "space cadet" but the seriousness of the situation must be borne in mind. Friends are generally willing to verify the patient's drug use and offer that "This time he really overdid it."A drug screen is helpful in retrospect but of little help in the acute management phase. The clinical picture is further complicated by the fact that many street drugs are impure, cut with other agents or are not even the type thought to have been purchased by the patient.

The use of a few milligrams of amphetamine orally over months for dieting produces a second clinical picture. Usually, patients are not aware of the possible dangers of this situation. Frequently, their physicians are equally unaware of the problems and in some instances do not want to be aware of the complications.

These patients have a curbing of their appetites, but when the pills are discontinued there is usually a rebound of their appetites. The appearance of the so-called "munchies" frequently results in the patients "having" to start on the amphetamines once again. In terms of the simplified model of amphetamine action, this chronic use of amphetamines "overworks" the dopamine system and eventually it can become "depleted." At this point, when the patient stops the amphetamines, there is the likelihood of developing symptoms of a primary affective disorder.

They become lethargic, despondent and display psychomotor retardation. Clearly, the situation for chronic addiction is ripe. It should be noted that amphetamines are not *antidepressants* but are "uppers" or "crispers." They have no place in the treatment of primary affective disorders. The main point is that the symptom of depression is not pathognomonic of the depressive phase of a primary affective disorder.

The third presentation of amphetamine abuse occurs when the patient titrates his amphetamine dose to avoid the toxic "high," though in excess of the diet suppression requirements. In a few months, he may develop a paranoid state which is very difficult to clinically differentiate from functional schizophrenia. In essence, the dopamine system has been chronically "turned on" but not acutely flooded or chronically depleted.

This last presentation leads to amphetamine being proposed as a chemical model for schizophrenia, a so-called Model Psychosis. The question is whether there has been a *de novo* creation of the psychosis by the drug or an unmasking of a premorbid substrate of schizophrenia. Some studies suggest that it is not an unmasking, since the patients had no suggestion of schizophrenia prior to taking the amphetamine. In the clinical setting, the problem is compounded by the fact that as many as half of the patients had indications of a functional problem prior to use of the drug.

The neuroleptic drugs, such as the phenothiazines, are effective in reversing the clinical picture seen with dopamine release due to amphetamine. This works by virtue of their ability to block postsynaptic dopamine receptors. In many cases, the outcome is a partial defect state of overall mental functioning. It is a constant source of amazement that people who may be resistant to taking prescribed medications will take a pill from a "friend" without knowing what is contains. Equally unusual is the fact that some physicians still maintain that "uppers" can be prescribed with little chance of abuse because they are not physiologically addictive in low doses.

Although the biochemical aspects of the schizophrenic process continue to be elusive, the work done on therapeutic agents has been of great importance in defining the clinical syndrome. The success of these agents in treatment has been enormous and has had a truly revolutionary impact on psychiatry.

PSYCHOLOGICAL THEORIES

It is helpful to begin this discussion by briefly outlining some aspects of psychoanalytic theory. Some points were mentioned earlier.

The *psychosexual* or *libidinal model* relates to the normal development of the mind as a progression through a series of age-specific stages. Each stage has characteristic mental processes which result in a particular organization of mental functioning. The mental processes associated with each stage become progressively less primitive as the mind matures.

Each stage of the psychosexual model has associated with it particular mental conflicts. Normal development will have resolution of these conflicts. At subsequent stages these conflicts will be renewed and reworked by the more mature mental processes.

In the first five years of life, three stages are negotiated. These are the oral, anal and phallic stages. Successful completion of these early stages is crucial. Flaws in the maturation processes incurred in these early phases can be the focus for abnormal mental functioning in adulthood.

By early adulthood, the primitive mental processes should have been replaced by mature processes. Reemergence of processes used in early functioning but normally replaced with maturation indicates that *regression* has taken place. Schizophrenia can be viewed as a severe regression in mental functioning and domination of the mental state by primitive processes. The regression is considered to be facilitated by mental stress in a setting of malresolution or incomplete resolution having occured in the first stage of psychosexual development.

This concept stresses that "the child is father to the man." Examples of schizophrenic symptoms which reflect the reemergence of primitive processes such as autism have been discussed earlier.

The *topographical model* considers the mind to be made up of three interacting units which are the *unconscious*, the *preconscious* and the *conscious*. The unconscious material persists with a mental representation of primitive processes. The conscious mind uses mature secondary processes and the primitive primary processes are excluded in the unperturbed mental functioning.

Slips of the tongue, so-called parapraxis, is an example of a momentary breakthrough of primary processes from the unconscious into the conscious mind. There has been a momentary "relaxation" of the censoring function of the preconscious mind.

During sleep, the censoring function is reduced and primary process material emerges into the conscious mind in the form of dream content. The content of dreams is a partial expression of unconscious material and its analysis offers a "royal highway" to the unconscious mind.

The emergence of primary process into the conscious mind during the awakened state indicates a perturbation of the mental state. In schizophrenia, the mental perturbation is so severe that there is a significant and sustained invasion of the conscious unit by primitive processes.

The *structural* or *tripartite model* proposes that the mind is made up of three interacting components which are the *id*, the *ego* and the *superego*. The id is unconscious and its organization is in terms of primitive primary process. The id deals with the mental representation of instinctual drives and response patterns. These drives and responses demand instant gratification and lack restraint, since this would require secondary processes for its imposition. The superego is primarily unconscious. It is made up of a set of sanctions incorporated during the developmental process, in particular those imposed during the resolution of the phallic stage of the psychosexual model. In this sense, the superego acts as a "governor" for the interacting tripartite units.

The ego has both conscious and unconscious components. The conscious component is made up of mature secondary processes which include features such as language and memory, concepts of ordering, time and space, as well as mobility and behavioural functions. Important features of the unconscious part of the ego are the *defense mechanisms.*

Intrapsychic conflicts are common. These can be produced in the conscious and the unconscious mental compartments. The primitive process drives with their "all and now" gratification demands pose a constant potential threat to aspects of the conscious ego. The maintenance of intrapsychic equilibrium between the interacting units is a function of the unconscious ego defense mechanisms. The impetus of the drives has to be kept but conscious ego functions have to be protected and the superego sanctions respected.

The need to employ specific unconscious defense mechanisms in a pathological manner to maintain intrapsychic equilibrium leads to the characteristic symptoms of the *neuroses*. In general, the resultant mental distortion does not have the severity associated with the psychoses. For example, the use of the unconscious defense mechanism of displacement results in the features of a phobia whilst the pathological employment of conversion can give rise to a conversion hysteria.

The defense mechanisms of the schizophrenic patient are unable to containt the psychic turmoil. Primitive ego defense mechanisms reflect more directly in the mental functioning and the conscious ego functions are severely compromised. The overall *ego integrity* is markedly distorted and symptoms including hallucinations, delusions and formal thought disorders arise.

It is worthwhile recalling the "need versus fear" concept. The individual has a necessity to maintain equilibrium among the three components of the structural model. Distortion of the conscious aspects of the ego occurs in the attempt to restore a balance to the dynamic equation. Such a "solution" involves *distortion of the ego boundaries* with a subsequent adjustment in the concept of "reality."

The principal psychoanalytic models were formulated in sequence to account for clinical observations. They have a number of common threads and areas of overlap. Early childhood development is identified as the key to adult mental stability. The analytic theories stress that flaws or failure of resolution of intrapsychic conflicts in the early developmental states can act as the focus for adulthood regression.

The primitiveness of the schizophrenic process is stressed in all three models. Regression results in the re-emergence of primitive processes into the conscious mind and the employment of primitive ego defense mechanisms in an attempt to maintain the dynamic mental equilibrium.

Other psychological models of schizophrenia have been developed as extrapolations from theories of personality. In general, other personality or analytic theories maintain the principles of the classical psychoanalytic theory.

The *Radical Ego* model of schizophrenia proposes that instead of a regression to primitive processes, the disorder is due to failure to move beyond primary process thinking. This suggests the pathology is a failure to reach a mature pattern rather than regression to earlier processes of mental functioning.

Erickson's stages of psychosexual development span the whole life cycle rather than focusing on the early phase. There are a number of similarities with the classical psychoanalytic model. Erickson describes the first few years of life as characterised by a struggle to develop trust or non-trust. The failure to establish concepts of trust predisposes to the use of projection as a means of coping with intrapsychic conflict. As in the classical psychoanalytic model, paranoid features imply psychosexual developmental problems in the early stage.

Like Erickson, the *Psychobiology* model of Meyer lessens the focus on the early years and stresses the need for a whole life history in the formulation of mental disorders. Meyer emphasises the need to view the patient as a whole. He used the term *paragasia* to describe patients with schizophrenia. The *Interpersonal* model of Sullivan stresses the need to view development of mental functioning throughout the entire life cycle. In particular, Sullivan looks at behaviour as a means of dealing with others and not primarily determined by unconscious intrapsychic processes. This need to consider the entire development and the ongoing interpersonal interactions as evidenct of pathology is summed up in Sullivan's phrase "Man is an act not a fact." The early infant experiences are undifferentiated in what Sullivan referred to as the *prototaxic* mode. This mode, with its lack of concepts such as self and non-self, occurs in the schizophrenic disorder.

There are many psychological theories for schizophrenia but until the disorder is more fully understood, their validity cannot be adequately tested.

SOCIOLOGICAL THEORIES

Mental illness has been defined as difficulties with authority and with maintenance of interpersonal relationships. All illness produces a distortion in sociological terms. For this reason, one must approach any clinical problem with consideration of biological, psychological and sociological factors.

Social distortions can produce mental symptoms which are similar to those of the psychoses. However, even when a disorder is associated with clear sociological problems at the presentation, care must be exercised before concluding the sociological factors are etiological. Regardless of the etiology, the sociological factors are critical in regard to the outcome.

Much has been written about sociological factors and family dynamics as a possible etiology of schizophrenia. It has been proposed that schizophrenia is the result of chaotic family interactions. It is true that the family of the schizophrenic generally has pathological modes of interpersonal exchanges. Two points must be considered.

Firstly, it is possible that the chaotic family interactions are a result, not the cause, of having a family member who is schizophrenic. The sociological perturbation is then the result of schizophrenia rather than its etiology.

Secondly, schizophrenia patients "producing" schizophrenic children may do so not because of distorted family interactions but simply because they pass a genetic disorder on to their children.

Particular family interaction patterns stressed in connection with schizophrenia include the view that the child has to learn pathological modes of mental functioning to survive in an environmental chaos during a critical period of developoment. This is a "need versus fear" model in which pathological functioning brings some consistency and order to the maturation period. This is more basic than simply assuming that the psychosis is learned aberrant behaviour.

Another construct concerns particular family constallations. The *schism* family is one that is divided into multiple "warring camps" which necessitates the child adopting pathological modes of coping during critical periods of development. In the *skew* family, the interactions, both psychological and physiological, are dominated by a disturbed family member who is never identified to the children as being ill.

Some theorists point to a characteristic *communication deviance* in the family of schizophrenics. Although there is communication, it lacks cognitive clarity. In the critical early phase of mental development, pathological processes are adopted. It is said that the combination of genetic predisposition to schizophrenia and communication deviance greatly increases the likelihood of schizophrenia. The presence of communication deviance alone predisposes only to schizotypal disorders.

The term *double bind* is used to describe a type of pathological interaction between parent and child. Again, there is the notion of induced distortions during a critical phase of development. This child is exposed to verbal messages coupled with contradictory verbal or non-verbal messages. The parent says, "That is perfectly all right with me," but does so with a look of resigned displeasure as she turns away from the child. The double bind is repeatedly administered and the child is in no position to escape the interactions.

The focus of the developmental theories of schizophrenia is the mother, since she is usually the dominant character in the early development phase. The *schizophrenogenic* mother is described as one unable to provide the necessary psychological and physiological mothering in the critical developmental phase. Instead, the child is exposed to one of the deviant modes described above.

It is clear that these deviant modes are seen in the histories of schizophrenics but many children exposed to such modes do not go on to develop schizophrenia. They are not exclusive to schizophrenia and occur in a range of mental disorders. Also, there are schizophrenics who do not give a development history which cites such family interactions. The non-specificity places an etiological role in great doubt.

Once the schizophrenic process presents, there is invariably a distortion of social parameters resulting in a range of secondary symptoms and difficulties. The importance of these sociological problems cannot be overemphasized in terms of treatment of the schizophrenias but may be overstated, particularly with hindsight, in terms of etiology.

CHAPTER 8

STATISTICS AND GENETICS OF THE SCHIZOPHRENIAS

Information of a statistical and genetic nature aids the investigation and clarification of an illness. Also, it helps in planning health care delivery. The compiling of such information is a difficult task. The data is a function of the design of the study: for example, the characteristics of the study's catchment area, the sampling techniques to identify subjects and the diagnostic inclusion and exclusion criteria applied in the study. Despite these factors there is a consistency in the findings from studies of schizophrenia. The following outlines some of the classical findings.

There is a characteristic *age of risk* for the first hospitalization due to schizophrenia. This is schematically shown in the following figure.

Figure 16

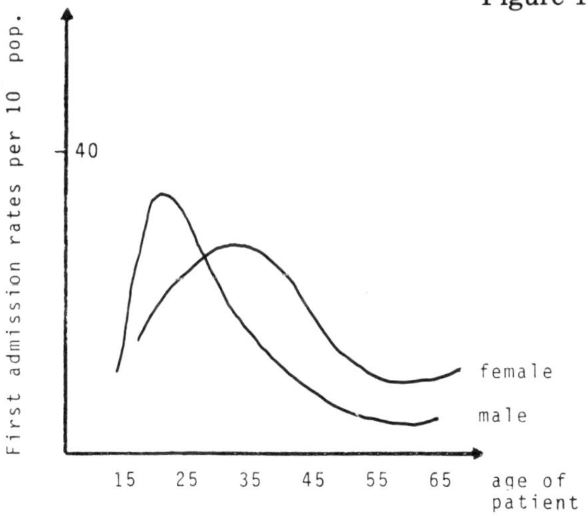

The risk is maximum between 15 and 45 years of age. There is a difference for the sexes. Men are at maximum risk between 15 and 25 years of age and women, between the ages of 25 and 35. Both sexes have an increase in risk beginning in the late 60's corresponding to the paraphrenic subgroup. A woman with schizophrenia is more likely to have married and to have become a parent prior to the first admission than is a schizophrenic man, because of the later age of onset and marriage at a younger age.

The total number of first admissions per year for schizophrenia is relatively consistent both over time and the country in which the study is carried out. In the following table, rounded-off figures are given for schizophrenia along with those of other major psychiatric disorders for comparison.

Admissions per year per 100,000 population		
	male	female
the schizophrenias	26	29
major affective disorders	14	24
others	44	88

Table 1

The schizophrenias are by no means the commonest admissions to psychiatric hospitals. However, schizophrenia accounts for the greatest single diagnosis of the chronically hospitalized patients. The admissions for schizophrenia are equal for men and women which is not the case for the other two disorders listed above.

An important statistic is the incidence of schizophrenia. Studies indicate that the incidence, that is to say the number of new cases that develop within the catchment area, is approximately 0.6 per thousand population. The incidence of all mental disorders is some 8 per thousand population which means that schizophrenia represents less than 8 percent of the total mental disorders in a community.

The prevalence, that is to say, the combined number of new and chronic cases within the catchment area, of schizophrenia is some 2 per thousand population. The prevalence of all mental disorders within a population has been reported as high as 80 percent but the majority of these conditions are not psychoses nor even require formal intervention by clinicians. It must be stressed that schizophrenia is a relatively rare condition. However, the diagnosis is applied to a much greater number of individuals than is warranted.

Information regarding the genetics of schizophrenia can be obtained by studying the risk of schizophrenia in the relatives of schizophrenics. The risk of an individual, whether man or woman, developing schizophrenia at some point in his lifetime with a negative family history for the disorder is approximately 1 percent. The risk for relatives of a schizophrenic, the so-called index case, is given in the following table.

```
Negative Family History

lifetime risk of becoming an index case 1%

Positive Family History

index case's child's lifetime risk 12%
index case's sibling's lifetime risk 8%
index case's parent's lifetime risk 5%
index case's uncle/stepsibling's risk 2%

both parents having schizophrenia places
the offspring's lifetime risk at 35/45%
```

Table 2

As can be seen, a positive family history significantly increases the risk. The relative at greatest risk is the offspring of the index case and the risk is equal for sons and daughters. The risk decreases as the relation to the index cases "weakens" and, significantly, step-siblings approach the general risk of 1 percent.

If both parents are schizophrenic, their offspring's risk of manifesting the disorder at some point during its lifetime is more than double that with a single affected parent.

Additional genetic information can be obtained from twin studies. Schizophrenic concordance rates are much higher for monozygotic twins then for dizygotic twins. The rate is some 60 percent for monozygotic and approximately 5 percent for dizygotic twins. Interestingly, though for obvious reasons the number of cases are rare, the concordance rates indicate similar trends if the twins are raised apart from birth.

Adoption studies are particularly valuable. In addition to indicating genetic characteristics, they shed light on the question of nature versus nurture in the development of schizophrenia. Children born to a schizophrenic mother but adopted at birth and raised by non-schizophrenic parents have a risk of developing schizophrenia similar to that of an offspring raised by its parents, one of whom is schizophrenic. Children born to non-schizophrenic couples but adopted at birth and raised by non-schizophrenics had a risk of developing schizophrenia the same as people with a negative family history for the disorder. This type of information points to the strong influence of biological factors in the nature-nurture equation for the etiology of schizophrenia.

Analysis of the genetic data is a complex problem and the indications at present are a polygenetic transmission of an autosomal recessive type with variable penetrance.

CHAPTER 9

TREATMENT OF THE SCHIZOPHRENIAS

The schizophrenias can be treated but not cured. It is important to distinguish between treatment and cure when discussing any medical disorder. The symptoms of schizophrenia in many cases can be eradicated or alleviated so that the patient can function in society.

The treatment of any clinical disorder, whether schizophrenia or a broken hip, should be approached under these headings, namely, biological, psychological and sociological. The pinning of a broken hip is only one aspect of treatment and in many cases it turns out to be a minor feature of the patient's overall recovery.

SOCIOLOGICAL TREATMENT

Schizophrenia is not experienced in a vacuum. The simple act of hospitalization may both help and hinder the situation. The removal of a patient from the community or family setting often eases the symptoms to a marked degree. Hospitalization may result in family regrouping or closing its ranks to exclude the patient which makes eventual discharge back to the family problematic.

From the onset, the family must be assisted in its understanding of the problems. In many instances, the patient's relatives experience guilt for having "caused" or "greatly contributed" to the schizophrenia. Certainly, any notions they have about the disorder being untreatable or necessarily requiring chronic care must be removed.

A prolonged hospitalization may result in the patient's developing an *institutional syndrome* with loss of initiative and self-responsibility. Such social regression by the patient makes a successful return to the community very difficult in spite of alleviation of the presenting symptoms.

The hospital *milieu* has little to no effect on the alleviation and treatment of the primary rank symptoms of schizophrenia. It has not been shown that a *therapeutic milieu* influences the first rank symptoms to any discernible degree. However, the "snake pit" hospital milieu promotes detrimental habit formations and features of the regressive institutional syndrome.

The sociological conditions to which patients are discharged has a definite influence on the overall outcome for schizophrenia. In general, facilities for schizophrenics in the community are pathetically inadequate and this frequently contributes to a deteriorative "revolving door" situation.

The contribution of social workers to the successful treatment of schizophrenia cannot be overemphasized. They have a role involving the patients and their families in regards to secondary symptomatology and discharge planning.

PSYCHOLOGICAL TREATMENT

Psychotherapy has a role in the treatment of a schizophrenic and often is more effective when directed to involve members of the patient's family.

There is little, if indeed any, evidence that insight or psychoanalytic psychotherapy has an effect on the removal of primary symptoms of schizophrenia. Supportive psychotherapy, both individual and in the form of groups, is helpful during inpatient and outpatient phases of treatment.

The role of psychotherapy is more apparent in the resolution phase of schizophrenia, particularly in dealing with the secondary symptoms of schizophrenia. It is the supportive rather than insight form of psychotherapy which is most useful in preventing relapses as measured by the need for rehospitalization. Nevertheless, studies show that relapse rates for placebo treated patients and those given only psychotherapy, of any form, differ marginally. Also, the relapse rates for patients who receive drugs only and those who receive drugs and psychotherapy do not differ significantly.

BIOLOGICAL TREATMENT

If the patient is correctly diagnosed, if the intervention is early in the course of the disorder, if the "malignancy" of the disorder is not overwhelming, if the biological treatment is given correctly and if the patient complies, then such treatment is effective in most cases of schizophrenia. This statement is supported by numerous controlled studies.

The principal biological or somatic therapies are psychotropic drugs and electroconvulsive therapy (ECT). All clinicians ought to be aware of the effectiveness of antipsychotic medications in the management and treatment of many organic psychoses encountered in all specialties. Furthermore, most primary care physicians will have occasion to treat remitted schizophrenics receiving drug therapy.

Electroconvulsive therapy is indicated in the treatment of certain subtypes of schizophrenia. Its principal indication is in the treatment of catatonic schizophrenia of both the agitated and retarded forms. Indeed, ECT is the treatment of choice in catatonic schizophrenia. There is evidence of effectiveness in the acute phase of schizophrenia and in the non-nuclear schizophrenias of schizophreniform and brief reactive psychoses. There is little indication of effectiveness in the treatment of the other nuclear schizophrenias, namely paranoid and hebephrenic, or in chronic schizophrenia. This somatic therapy has less contraindications and associated side effects than psychotropic drugs but is not practical in long term maintenance treatment.

Psychotropic drugs became generally available in the sixties and brought about a revolution in the treatment of the schizophrenias. These drugs allowed other treatment modes, such as the psychological and sociological, a better opportunity to be effectively applied as adjunct therapies.

Before discussing these medications, it is helpful to review some neurotransmitter biochemistry. This discussion will be limited to three neurotransmitters, namely, the catecholamines *dopamine* and *norepinephrine* and the indolamine *serotonin.*

These neurotransmitters do not cross the *blood brain barrier* but are synthesized within the central nervous system from precursors which can cross the barrier. These precursors are tyrosine for the catecholamines and tryptophan for serotonin. The synthesis of these neurotransmitters is shown in the following figure.

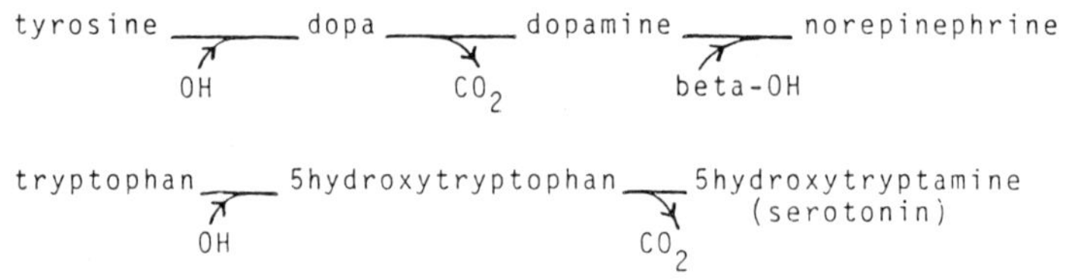

Figure 17

The mode of action of the antipsychotic or *neuroleptic* drug can be illustrated by focusing on one neurotransmitter, namely dopamine, applied to a single synapse model. This is a great oversimplification for a matter so complex as brain chemistry but the model serves the present discussion. The "life cycle" of a dopamine unit is schematically outlined in the following figure.

Dopamine is synthesized in the pre-synaptic terminal from a tyrosine precursor and stored in vesicles to await release into the synaptic cleft. The site of action of the dopamine after release is a dopamine receptor located on the post-synaptic membrane. Occupation of this receptor by dopamine activates adenyl cyclase located in this membrane which in turn activates cyclic-AMP within the post-synaptic terminal. In this manner, the neuronal transmission has been completed from the pre-synaptic to the post-synaptic cell.

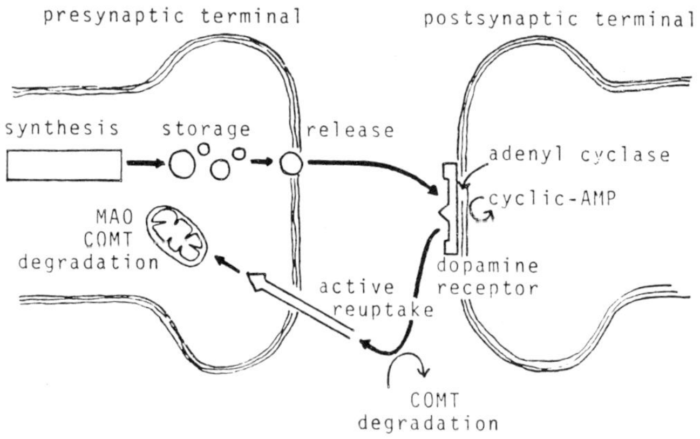

Figure 18

The principal breakdown of dopamine takes place in the pre-synaptic terminal via monoamine oxidase (MAO) and catechol-o-methyl transferase (COMT) enzymes. It is recalled that COMT is found in the synaptic cleft and was suggested as the enzyme involved in the transmethylation hypothesis of schizophrenia. Since the principal breakdown occurs presynaptically, the neurotransmitter must undergo an active reuptake across the pre-synaptic membrane from the synaptic cleft after its release from the post-synaptic receptor.

The mode of action of the neuroleptics can be summarized as an ability to occupy post-synaptic dopamine receptors. The neuroleptics are in competition with dopamine for these sites. At any point in time, these post-synaptic receptors are variously unoccupied or locked into either a neuroleptic or a neurotransmitter.

The ability of the drug to compete with the neurotransmitter for receptor occupation appears to be a necessary property in order for it to be clinically effective inthe treatment of schizophrenia. If the structure of the neuroleptic is altered so that this receptor affinity is lost, then the clinical effectiveness disappears. It does not necessarily follow that the greater the receptor blocking ability the greater the clinical effectiveness. As mentioned previously, this discussion concerns a simple model and it is a giant step from a receptor to a neuropsychiatric disorder.

The blockade of the post-synaptic receptor by the neuroleptic produces a "chain reaction." The post-synaptic receptor and terminal is now "starved" of dopamine and the result is a step-up of dopamine production in the pre-synaptic terminal. This is indicated by the increased activity of tyrosine hydroxylase which is the rate limiting enzyme in dopamine synthesis.

The seizure threshold in this synaptic model is defined in terms of the percentage of post-synaptic dopamine receptors at a given point in time occupied by dopamine. The neuroleptics, as a result of competition with dopamine for the receptors, lower the seizure threshold. These drugs are thus *epileptogenic* and relate to the term neuroleptic being applied to them.

In view of the apparent relationship between some features of epilepsy and some psychotic symptoms, it is interesting that medications which effectively treat schizophrenia are epileptogenic. It should be noted that the use of controlled seizures by electroconvulsive methods (ECT) is therapeutic for some subtypes of schizophrenia.

The analeptic drugs, such as amphetamine, can closely mimic the symptoms of schizophrenia. They effectively flood the post-synaptic receptor by promoting the synthesis and release of dopamine from the pre-synaptic terminal and decreasing the breakdown of the neurotransmitter. The flooding action raises the seizure threshold of the synaptic unit.

The risk of neuroleptics inducing generalised seizures is low. Even in patients with pre-existing convulsive disorders, the induction of manifest seizures is rare. Seizures tend to occur in patients who have a sudden and notable increase in neuroleptic dosage or when beginning treatment.

Although neuroleptic agents reach the brain via the blood supply and are distributed throughout the brain, there is a *site specificity* as regards their mode of action. As a comparison, the antibiotic treatment of a brain abcess involves delivery of the drug to the brain as a whole but the action is site specific to the region of the abcess. For neuroleptics, the site specificity in the treatment of schizophrenia involves the limbic system. Therapeutic differences of the neuroleptics may be related to differences in their affinity for these sites.

The differences in side effects associated with the various neuroleptics is related to their affinity for particular regions in the brain. These differences help in the selection of a particular neuroleptic. For example, an agent with low affinity for the corpus striatum but retaining affinity for the limbic system would be preferred in the treatment of a schizophrenic who had accompanying parkinsonism.

Clinicians, on the basis of experience, frequently have a preference for particular neuroleptics. Often, this is because their patients have responded well to a particular agent or more likely because they have had therapeutic failures on other neuroleptics. Sometimes these experiences lead to the erroneous conclusion that a specific neuroleptic is indicated in a particular subgroup of schizophrenia. The important point is that if the various neuroleptics are given equivalent therapeutic trials there is little difference in their ability to alleviate the primary symtoms of schizophrenia. The critical point is to be sure that the neuroleptic has an adequate therapeutic trial.

There are a number of steps the neuroleptic passes through between administration and excretion. These steps vary from patient to patient and neuroleptic to neuroleptic. For some steps, such as liver metabolism, the idiosyncracies are very marked and it is not at all surprising that a particular patient will have a therapeutic failure on one agent but not on another. It is difficult to be sure that a given drug has had a therapeutic trial.

Probably, the major factor in choosing between the various neuroleptics is the associated side effects. All medications have side effects and these vary in frequency and severity from patient to patient. Some side effects can be clinically advantageous. The hypnotic effect in addition to the dopamine receptor blockade can be an advantage in the management of a hyperactive patient or one with insomnia. On the other hand, a propensity for uptake in the corpus striatum can result in extrapyramidal side effects in addition to the desired receptor blockade, which is a disadvantage in treatment of the schizophrenic.

The choice of a particular neuroleptic is based on three points. Firstly, can an adequate dose of the drug be administered to the patient to alleviate the primary symptoms as quickly as possible? Secondly, are there any associated effects of the particular neuroleptic which could be advantageous in the management of this particular patient? Thirdly, what are the relative complications associated with the particular neuroleptic?

There are a number of "rules of thumb" which can be applied to the amount of drug given to the patient. It is often true that geriatrics have slower metabolism of neuroleptics as compared to younger patients. The crucial metabolism of these drugs by the microsomal enzymes in the liver is relatively impaired in the elderly. A "rule of thumb" is that the elderly require lower doses of neuroleptics for therapeutic effects. Similarly, patients with impaired liver function or those taking other medications which are metabolyzed by the liver system may require lower dosage of neuroleptics.

Another "rule of thumb" for dose requirement is that it can be adjusted on a milligram-per-kilogram body weight basis. Given the overall complexities of the pharmacology of neuroleptics and the marked idiosyncracies in pharmacokinetics, such rules are simply guides. It is tragic to see a patient given homeopathic therapy because of rigid adherence to a "rule of thumb" and equally tragic if a patient receives unnecessarily high doses leading to toxic side effects.

There are "typical" doses of neuroleptics but first it is necessary to review the major neuroleptic subtypes.

1. Phenothiazines

There are three principal subgroups within the phenothiazine subtype. These are the aliphatic, piperidine and piperazine compounds. Their structures are schematically shown in the following figure.

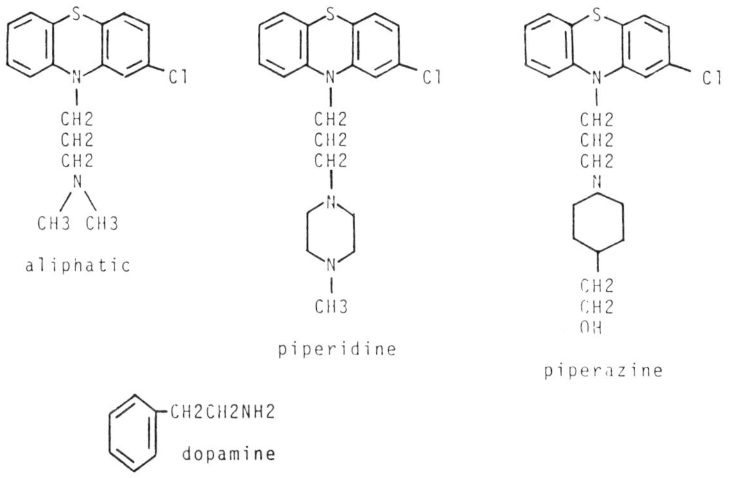

Figure 19

The similarities of structure involve a triple ring and a three carbon chain between successive nitrogen units. For comparison the schematic structure of dopamine is given.

2. Thioxanthenes

Again, the triple ring is present and the principal difference from the phenothiazines is the substitution of a double bonded carbon for a nitrogen unit.

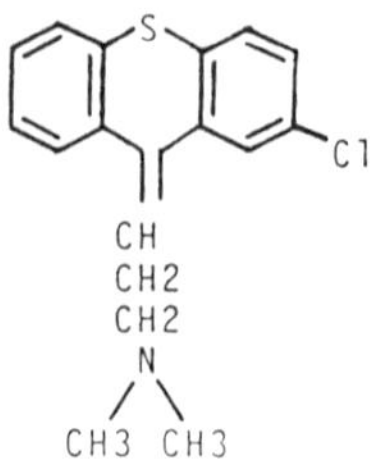

Figure 20

3. Butyrophenones

The structure of this neuroleptic subtype is fundamentally different from the phenothiazines and thioxanthenes. The primary example of this subtype, haloperidol, is schematically shown below.

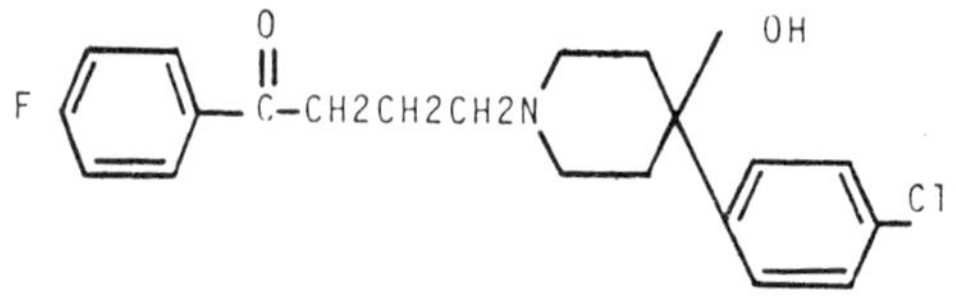

Figure 21

The following table lists some of the more commonly used neuroleptics and the typical oral dosage for use in the treatment of psychoses. Associated side effects and properties of clinical significance, namely, sedative effect, hypotensive effect, anticholinergic effects and extrapyramidal effects are graded according to frequency and severity.

In general terms the intramuscular route of administration provides higher serum levels over the oral route by some fifty percent except for the butyrophenone agent where absorption is approximately equal for the two routes of administration.

	mg per day	sedation	hypo-BP	antichol	EPS
Phenothiazine					
aliphatic chlorpromazine (Thorazine)	100-1500	marked	marked	marked	intermed
piperidine thioridazine (Mellaril)	100-800	marked	marked	marked	low
piperazine trifluperazine (Stelazine)	10-60	low	low	low	marked
Thioxanthene					
thiothixine (Navane)	10-60	low	low	low	intermed
Butyrophenone					
haloperidol (Haldol)	5-60	low	low	low	marked

Table 3

As was stressed earlier, the "rules of thumb" concerning age and body weight are guides as is the data given in the preceding table. The critical question in the clinical setting is how much and which neuroleptic to give to a particular patient.

Consider a patient, age thirty, with an acute schizophrenic breakdown manifested by florid first rank symptoms including marked motor agitation. The neuroleptic chlorpromazine (CPZ) would be a good selection since it can be given intramuscularly and has in addition to antipsychotic properties an initial hypnotic action clinically useful in this case.

The patient may be an idiosyncratic responder to neuroleptics and the key to medicating is to *titrate* the drug over time. A suitable set of orders might be *100mg po q2h prn* or *50mg im q2h prn.* The point is not so much the dosage given but the spacing between administrations and that additional doses are given according to need rather than passage of time alone. The criteria as to when available doses are repeated depends on the amelioration of symptoms and the degree of sedation of the patient. If, on the basis of the clinical picture, a faster titration is required, then the dosage can be maintained but the interval between possible administrations can be decreased. In the less florid cases, the interval can be prolonged using the same dosage.

The titration method "tailors" the drug therapy to the physiological and psychological needs of the patient. It is a more rational and safer method than applying generalizations in treatment. One gives as much medication as the clinical picture warrants bearing in mind the side effects of the neuroleptic and the relative contraindictions.

Side effects such as induced postural hypotension need to be monitored during the titration procedure. Also, the possible production of extrapyramidal symptoms should be borne in mind.

After twenty-four hours, a required daily dosage can be calculated. In cases of acute psychosis it is often better to continue the titration method for another day or so since the patient's psychosis may be escalating and the first day's total dose might be insufficient on following days. It is equally possible that on the second day the patient's mental state has improved and the first day's total dose may not be necessary.

In a geriatric patient presenting with the same symptoms, the dosage can be reduced by a factor of two but the same titration technique can be applied. Using chlorpromazine in such a patient would require particular attention to hypotensive problems.

A pattern of required daily dose appear after a few days and this allows ordering the drug on a fixed basis. Since the halflife of the neuroleptics is typically in excess of twenty-four hours, a steady state plasma level should be established within a week or so. It is not necessary to give the drug in divided dosages through the day at this point in therapy. It may be that when medication is taken a transient, though significant, hypotensive episode occurs which is troublesome to the patient. In general, this is not a problem, especially after a week or so on an unchanging daily dose. The most convenient time for the single administration of the total daily dose is in the evening. It may well be that overall compliance is better under these circumstances since patients often forget to take medications during the working day and the family can remind patients to take the night time regimen.

Florid symptoms make titration easier since one adjusts titration to obvious features of the disturbed mental state. In the case of chronic schizophrenia, titration is more difficult since the symptoms are frequently less apparent and their changes occur more slowly. Information from old medical records about drug dose and type of neuroleptic is particularly helpful. The changes in dose may be made at intervals of days rather than hours.

It is important, both in acute and chronic schizophrenia, to recognise that adequate therapeutic trials require sufficient time as well as dosage. As a rule, the duration of a therapeutic trial involving adequate dosage should run two to three weeks before that agent is discontinued and another type of neuroleptic is instituted. Quickly changing from one neuroleptic to another is self defeating.

There is little or no advantage in using neuroleptic "cocktails." All one is doing by combining two or more neuroleptics is mixing their therapeutic properties and their associated side effects. When improvement occurs or changes are required, it is unclear which drug is responsible. It is far more rational to increase the dose of a single neuroleptic as part of a therapeutic trial.

In some cases, the hypnotic and sedation properties of some neuroleptics is a disadvantage. A less sedative neuroleptic such as haloperidol may be the choice in this situation. The lack of drowsiness may make the assessment of the drug's effect on the primary symptoms a simpler task. A suitable set of titration orders for haloperidol might be *10mg po q2h prn* or *10mg im q2h prn*. The intervals between doses can be adjusted depending on the clinical situation as discussed earlier.

Lack of associated drowsiness is useful in the treatment of toxic and organic psychoses. These patients frequently have impaired consciousness secondary to the toxic agents or the organic impairment and it is helpful to select a neuroleptic which does not add to this component of the impaired mental state.

There are combination drugs which contain a neuroleptic and an antidepressant in the same tablet. This type of drug should be avoided in the initial pharmacotherapy of patients. It is unclear which component is beneficial during treatment. There are cases which finally require a combination of psychotropic medications for maximum response. If a combination tablet is available with the correct ratio of drugs, then it could be substituted in the final phase of treatment.

Much has been written about *rapid tranquilisation*. This involves titration of neuroleptics at short time intervals between administrations. It should be made clear what is meant by the word tranquilisation. It is unfortunate that neuroleptics are often called *major tranquilisers* since they do not produce a tranquil state *per se*.

Rapid titration, with intervals between administration of twenty minutes or so, and sometimes involving intravenous delivery of the neuroleptic agent, may be necessary in the very disturbed patient. The end result is a hypnotic effect which might be tranquility for the medical staff, but not the patient. The real question should be whether rapid medicating of this type results in a more rapid lysis of the psychotic symptoms. This is possibly not the case. The clinical need to quickly control some patients who present a clear danger to themselves or others is probably the major indication for this method.

There is often a need to manage agitated patients during postoperative recovery or those with organic brain syndromes who are a danger to themselves. Neither of these situations need manifest psychotic symptoms. Titration of neuroleptics is to be preferred over such drugs as benzodiazepines or barbiturates since these latter agents frequently add to agitation and confusion of the patients.

A technique to manage these patients involves intravenous haloperidol. It should be recalled that this medication was introduced in Europe as an intravenous drug. A possible titration method consists of increasing dosage given at close fixed intervals. For example, 2.5 milligrams by intravenous "push" followed some 20 minutes later by 5.0 milligrams then 10 milligrams after a further 20 minutes and so on. This technique of rapid neuroleptic administration requires that the clinician "remain by the bedside" and be aware of the signs and symptoms of neurotoxic complications.

The geriatric patient with agitation and emotional lability generally deteriorates with the use of benzodiazepines and barbiturates. Even in the absence of psychotic symptoms, a suitable drug to treat the organic patient with primary anxiety is haloperidol, because of its lower incidence of drowsiness. It is important to begin titration with small doses such as 0.5mg per day. This can be increased on a daily basis with 0.5mg increments using the clinical symptoms as the guide. If the dosage gets to a range of 5 to 10mg per day without improvement, it is wise to reassess the case. It may well be that the disorder is one of agitated depression rather than an organic brain syndrome.

Low dose neuroleptics in the range of one tenth of the antipsychotic daily dose are useful anxiolytic agents. It is not necessary that the anxiety be related to an underlying psychosis. These agents do not present with the addiction problems associated with the more commonly used benzodiazepines. Twenty-five to fifty milligrams of thioridazine or chlorpromazine are excellent. At these doses it is unlikely that the patient will develop significant side effects in short term use.

For some patients, it is necessary to increase the dose of neuroleptics into the gram range to alleviate symptoms.

Daily requirements of two to three grams of chlorpromazine are seen in practice. It is important to bear this in mind when formulating a therapeutic trial.

The long acting depot neuroleptics, such as fluphenazine, have an advantage in terms of patient compliance. Following a single deep muscle injection, there is a release of the agent into the blood stream over a number of weeks. After some twenty-four hours, this release is approximately at a steady rate. There is not a significant "dumping" syndrome associated with this agent, that is to say, a week's worth of medication is not released in a single day, resulting in overdosing of the patient. There appears to be no advantage in doing an oral fluphenazine trial prior to beginning the depot form of the neuroleptic.

The early use of depot medication was for long term maintenance of chronic schizophrenics. At present, this form of neuroleptic is frequently used in the treatment of acute cases. A titration method against clinical symptoms can still be employed in prescribing this medication. A suitable initial dose is lcc which contains 25mg of the agent. In acute phases, this can be repeated after three or four days and a typical maintenance requirement is lcc weekly, or in some cases every two or three weeks, depending on the clinical picture.

At this point, it is appropriate to discuss in detail the side effects associated with the neuroleptics.

1. Dystonia

In as little as an hour or as long as weeks following the initiation of neuroleptic therapy, the patient can experience a dystonic reaction. The variability of onset and the wide range of dosage which can result in these reactions is a reflection of the idiosyncracies of these medications.

The acute dystonias are often dramatic and particularly frightening for the patient. The signs and symptoms of the severe cases include torticollis, trismus, ocular gyric crisis, opisthotonos, generalised hypertonicity in the limbs and panic.

The prompt administration of medications such as benztropine or benedryl will quickly reverse this side effect. Specifically, 2mg of benztropine given intramuscularly or 50mg of benedryl given intravenously will improve the situation within minutes.

The more common dystonias will be discussed along with the parkinsonian-like syndrome associated with the neuroleptics.

2. Parkinsonian-Like Syndrome and Extrapyramidal Symptoms

The classical problem of parkinsonism is a deficiency of dopamine at the basal ganglia (corpus striatum) because of insufficient synthesis of this neurotransmitter in the substantia nigra. The neuroleptics are taken up in the basal ganglia to varying degrees and are all dopamine blockers. Induction of a parkinsonian-like syndrome is to be expected. Sufficient dopamine is being delivered *via* the nigrastriatum tract but there has been a reduction in the available sites in the basal ganglia.

As can be seen from the previous table, the piperidine, thioridazine, has a low incidence of parkinsonian extrapyramidal problems. This is because of its low affinity for dopamine receptors located in the corpus striatum. The butyrophenone haloperidol has a high incidence of extrapyramidal side effects because of its great affinity for receptors in this region of the brain. The relative incidence of such problems is important in the choice of neuroleptics for certain patients.

The earliest clinical indication of neuroleptic-induced parkinsonism is usually a combination of *dystonia* and *akinesia.* The well known pill-rolling at rest hand tremor is a later finding inthe drug induced cases. In many cases of non-drug induced parkinsonism, the earliest indication is a poverty of motion which is frequently misinterpreted as fatigue or old age.

The increased muscle tone associated with extrapyramidal problems leads to a flexion of the arms and they no longer swing fluidly when the patient walks. There can be hypertonicity of the legs resulting in replacement of the normal stride by a shuffling gait of *petit marche*. This muscle rigidity produces a poverty of motion and features of akinesia. There are difficulties initiating a step and making quick changes in direction when walking. The patients compensate for these problems with a *festinating gait*. This is a characterised by short steps and a stooped posture with the person "chasing his centre of gravity." Often, this results in steady acceleration and difficulties in coming to a halt.

These early features of akinesia due to neuroleptics are often passed off as indications of depression, anergia or oppositionalism in the period prior to an obvious tremor.

A frequent sign of neuroleptic induced parkinsonism is *cogwheeling*. As the patient's arm is extended by the clinician, a ratchet-like effect can be palpated at the bicep tendon. This "catching" effect can also be demonstrated when the patient's wrist is slowly rotated by the examiner. This cogwheeling may be a reflection of the tremor associated with parkinsonism.

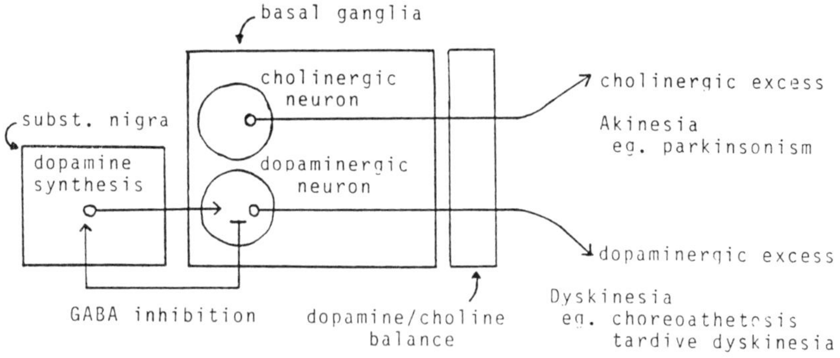

Figure 22

The normal functioning corpus striatum can be envisaged as a balanced systemof dopaminergic and cholinergic neurons. It is suggested that synthesis of dopamine in the substantia nigra is controlled by inhibitive feedback involving the neurotransmitter gamma-aminobutyric acid (GABA). The neuroleptics alter this balance by reducing the effectiveness of dopamine at the post-synaptic sites in the basal ganglia. This change results in the extra pyramidal symptoms and parkinsonism.

An alternative representation of the situation can be used to outline methods of treating extrapyramidal side effects and is shown in the following figure.

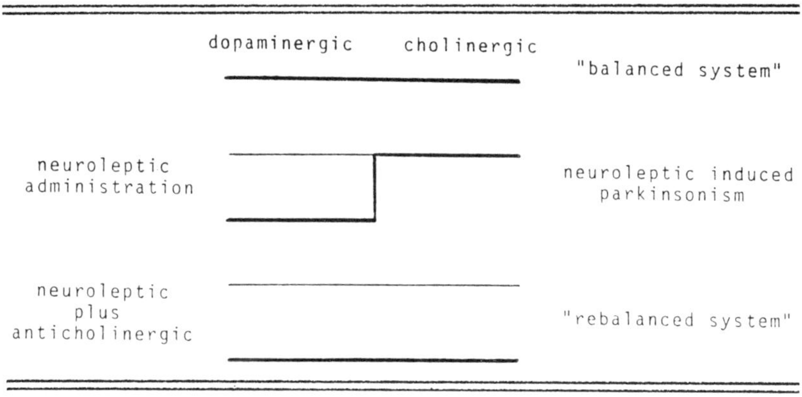

Figure 23

The imbalance due to the effective dopamine reduction by the neuroleptics can be removed by reduction of the cholinergic system. This can be done using anticholinergics such as benztropine or trihexyphenidyl. A frequent treatment is 2mg of benztropine orally two or three times per day.

The proposed mechanism of a 50mg intravenous bolus of the antihistamine benedryl restoring balance to this system is that it promotes dopamine effects by stimulation of cyclic-AMP.

In the case of non-drug induced parkinson akinesia, the drug levo-dopa, a precursor of dopamine, crosses the blood-brain-barrier and increases the brain synthesis of dopamine in the substantia nigra. Levo-dopa is not applicable to the treatment of neuroleptic induced parkinsonism.

The likelihood of a neuroleptic provoking extrapyramidal symptoms varies from patient to patient but is more likely for some of the neuroleptics. The occurence of these side effects is not clearly related to the neuroleptic dose. It is debatable whether anticholinergics, such as benztropine 2mg bid, should be given prophylactically with the commencement of neuroleptic therapy. For many patients, the occurrence of extrapyramidal side effects such as dystonia or akinesia is sufficiently upsetting that they refuse further neuroleptic treatment even if the side effect is quickly reversed.

The anticholinergic agents have their own side effects including dry mouth, blurred vision, constipation and difficulties with micturation. Therefore, it is best not to use the anticholinergics unless extrapyramidal side effects occur. In cooperative patients one can wait and see if such side effects develop but it should be remembered that they can develop weeks after the commencement of neuroleptic treatment. It has been said that as many as eighty percent of patients receiving neuroleptics are being unnecessarily given prophylactic anticholinergics.

In addition to akinesia, the neuroleptics can induce *akasthesia.* The patient becomes restless with pacing or standing on one spot and shifting of weight from one foot to the other. If akasthesia occurs soon after introduction to neuroleptics, it is frequently mistaken for increased anxiety and thought to be indicative for an increase in the neuroleptic dose. When akasthesia occurs after prolonged neuroleptic treatment, it may be mistaken as a sign of relapse and the neuroleptic dose increased. Anticholinergic agents similar to those mentioned earlier are the treatment for this neuroleptically-induced *dyskinesia.*

3. Anticholinergic Effects

The critical property of neuroleptics in the treatment of schizophrenia is their ability to block post-synaptic dopamine receptors. They also have additional anticholinergic effects to varying degrees across the various agents. These anticholinergic properties in general are unwanted complications.

These anticholinergic properties should not be confused with the need for anticholinergics to counteract possible extrapyramidal problems. As an illustration, thioridazine has a low incidence of extrapyramidal side effects not because of "built in" anticholinergic effects but because it has reduced dopamine blocking affinity within the basal ganglia.

It is almost invariable that patients receiving neuroleptics experience a dry mouth early in treatment. Sometimes, this is marked but other times the symptom is elicited only on direct questioning. The drymouth results from anticholinergic blockade of the parasympathetic innervation of the secretory components of the seventh and ninth cranial nerves.

In many cases, this effect diminishes after a week or so but in others the dry mouth persists. Reassurance of the patient that the occurrence does not indicate a "bad reaction" to the neuroleptic is helpful. If the patient has developed extrapyramidal symptoms requiring anticholinergic drugs, then this affect is enhanced.

Some patients have a problem with drooling rather than a dry mouth. This is often the case in non-drug related parkinsonism. The problem is due to laryngeal spasm, not production of excessive saliva. The salivation may actually be reduced but they have difficulty swallowing due to the laryngeal spasm and the saliva accumulates in the mouth.

The laryngeal spasm is an extrapyramidal effect and the only one which is not terminated during sleep. Patients frequently awaken with a damp pillow. In cases of acute dystonia, laryngeal spasm can be dramatic and frightening but anticholinergics will quickly reverse the problem.

Another early and frequent complaint due to neuroleptic anticholinergic properties is blurred vision due to *loss of accommodation*. This results from failure of the pupils to constrict during convergence. The patient's distant vision is unaffected but he cannot read print unless he holds the page at arm's length. Accommodation is mediated *via* the parasympathetic Edinger-Westphal nucleus located in the brain-stem. This problem will also be accentuated if the patient needs anticholinergic drugs to prevent neuroleptically induced extrapyramidal side effects. There is no treatment for this blurred vision and one hopes there will be sympathetic system adjustment during the course of neuroleptic treatment. In chronically treated patients, it is often necessary for them to have a change made in their spectacles or perhaps to begin using eye-glasses.

Sustained dilation of the pupils due to neuroleptic anticholinergic effects can impair intraoccular drainage, which can become a problem in patients with glaucoma. Unless glaucoma is particularly severe, this side effect is not a contraindication to the use of neuroleptics but only suggests periodic evaluation of intraoccular pressure.

Anticholinergic effects of the neuroleptics on the peripheral nervous system can lead to constipation and, rarely, a case of paralytic ileus. In general, the bowel difficulties can be treated with stool softeners. Problems with micturation are occasionally induced but acute urinary retention is rare. Prostatic hypertrophy is not a contraindiction to the use of neuroleptics.

Finally, with respect to the anticholinergic effects of the neuroleptics, it should be remembered that they can provoke a drug induced psychosis. Clearly, the risk is greater if the patient is also receiving anticholinergic agents for prophylasis against extrapyramidal effects. The induced psychosis is in the form of an acute organic brain syndrome characterised by delirium. The elderly patient is more susceptible to this problem.

4. Cardiovascular Effects

Orthostatic hypotension is a frequent side effect of the drugs, and the probable cause is alpha-adrenergic blockage. It is prudent to tell the patients of possible transient dizziness or syncopal episodes when standing up from a lying position or getting out of a hot bath. It is well to stress to the patients that these effects are not a "bad reaction" to the neuroleptic. In many cases, rapid tolerance for the hypotensive problem develops.

As with all side effects and therapeutic effects of the neuroleptics, there is much patient idiosyncracy. Although hypotensive episodes are more likely in the elderly, it is not rare to find a "young linebacker" who develops significant hypotension on a comparatively low dose of a neuroleptic while a "frail little granny" has no such problem while receiving the same dose of that agent.

In general, conservative measures such as lowering the head of the bed are adequate treatment. The necessity of volume expanders is rare but in a predisposed geriatric or cardiology patient this may be required. In these patients, it may be well to give the daily requirement of neuroleptic in divided doses through the day to avoid transient effects until the patient develops some degree of tolerance.

Relatively benign changes in the electrocardiogram are frequent. Most often they involve ST-segment alterations and prolongation of the PR, QRS and QT intervals. In general, neuroleptics do not produce the quinidine-like conduction blockades associated with tricyclic antidepressants.

Postoperative psychoses can be encountered particularly following cardiovascular surgery. The neuroleptics are preferred over benzodiazepines or barbiturates in the management of such cases. The butyrophenone, haloperidol, is felt by many to be the drug of choice because of its low cardiotoxic effect, low hypnotic effect and the possibility of intravenous titration. This is also true for the management of other postoperative psychosis.

5. Metabolic Changes

Weight gain, and to some degree an increase in appetite, occur with the use of neuroleptics. Glucose tolerance can be altered but not to any degree of concern. False positive pregnancy tests can be induced and menstrual irregularities can occur although the latter is most often the result of psychogenic stress.

Galactorrhea can be directly attributed to the dopamine blockade activity of the neuroleptics. As many as forty percent of patients receiving substantial doses of neuroleptics can have discharge from the breast if "milked" and some five percent spontaneously lactate. Prolactin release is inhibited through a dopaminergic system. The dopamine blocking ability of neuroleptics can be estimated by their elevation of serum prolactin. Neuroleptics cross the placenta and possible teratogenic effects must be considered when prescribing these agents to pregnant women. In some cases of anorexia nervosa with notable reduction in gonadotropin release, low dose neuroleptic use has been reported in stimulating release of these hormones, suggesting a similar dopamine-related system.

6. Skin Changes

Photosensitivity is not infrequent in patients treated with neuroleptics. The problem becomes more likely after prolonged treatment but acute sensitivity to the sun can occur. Usually, simple sunscreen agents are adequate prophylaxis.

A rare skin lesion occurring after long term and usually high dose neuroleptic use takes the form of a magenta coloured rash over the cheek bones. Biopsy of the lesion shows a melanin-like material. Melanin production normally is related to the pathway which synthesis the catecholamines.

7. Eye Changes

In addition to loss of accommodation and the acute induction of ocular gyric crises, the structures of the eye can be directly affected by neuroleptics.

Lens and corneal opacities with little or no effect on vision can occur after prolonged use of neuroleptics. This can be reversed after a period of weeks if the drug is discontinued. It is possible to produce irreversible retinitis pigmentosa and this is especially seen after long term therapy with the piperidine thioridazine in daily doses in excess of one gram. Unlike the opacities, this condition is difficult to identify on general examination. The patient is unlikely to complain of decreased visual acuity until the condition is well advanced.

8. Hematology Changes

The white cell, red cell and platelet counts are often reduced by neuroleptics. This is rarely significant to the point of having to discontinue the neuroleptic. As one would expect, a mild eosinophilia can be induced by these drugs in certain patients.

In rare cases, less than one per thousand, the reduction in the granulocytes can become a matter of concern. These patients, often elderly, tend to have a number of debilitating problems involving a number of organ systems. They tend to have a week or so of mild fever, pneumonitis and meningismus, then suddenly, perhaps over a matter of hours, their condition deteriorates and the cell count plummets to an agranular cytosis with the possibility of death.

9. Gastrointestinal Effects

As previously mentioned, there is the possibility of constipation and patients may have stomach upset and nausea from the neuroleptic. These features could well be a reflection of the psychological turmoil.

Approximately one in a thousand patients develops jaundice on neuroleptics. This is a direct, conjugated, polar hyperbilirubinemia due to changes in the biliary duct cells. The enzymes associated with the hepatic cells such as LDH and SGOT may not altered but alkaline phosphatase, specifically its isoenzyme 5'-nucleotidase, is elevated. The problem is reversed by stopping the neuroleptic and in many cases changing to another type of neuroleptic does not renew the problem.

10. Epileptogenic Effects

Neuroleptics lower the seizure threshold and patients receiving these medications infrequently have seizures usually of the tonic-clonic variety. The incidence of seizures directly attributable to neuroleptics is about one percent. One can become overly concerned about the seizure potential of these agents.

Severe cases of delirium tremens often presents with neuropsychiatric symptoms unmanageable with benzodiazepines. The neuroleptics can be highly effective and should not be withheld because of the concern about seizures. Similarly, the patient with a history of seizures and symptoms requiring neuroleptics can be given these agents. If necessary the neuroleptics can be given in conjunction with anticonvulsants.

11. Tardive Dyskinesia

A primary concern with prolonged use of neuroleptics is the induction of *tardive dyskinesia.* This syndrome develops typically after years of neuroleptic therapy. It is a dyskinesia with creation of abnormal movements rather than the loss of movements in the akinesia of parkinsonism.

The dyskinesia most often consists of a progressive involvement of the buccolingual and facial muscles. There may be repetitive writhing movements of the lips, tongue, cheeks, nose and eyelids. This condition is usually seen in the elderly. It is insidious in development and difficult to separate out from movement disorder simply related to aging. The incidence of tardive dyskinesia varies depending on the diagnostic inclusion criteria but may occur in ten percent of patients on long term neuroleptic therapy.

In its severe form, even drinking and chewing are difficult. There may be progression to involve the upper extremities suggesting extension of the dysfunction within the bulbar tracts. As with all movement disorders, the symptoms become worse under stress including examination by the clinician but lessen when the patient is alone and relaxed. Such features should not be classed as "hysterical symptoms."

Occasionally, a similar syndrome is seen in children and young adults. This occurs in a matter of weeks after the initiation of neuroleptic therapy. It is more likely to have upper limb involvement along with the buccolingual dysfunction than in adult tardive dyskinesia. In contrast to the adult condition, it is quickly reversed by discontinuation of the neuroleptic.

A model suggested for tardive dyskinesia involves damage of the post-synaptic dopamine receptor due to prolonged interaction with the neuroleptic. The post-synaptic receptor becomes "hypersensitive" to dopamine. This may be from distortion of the post-synaptic terminal or alteration in the number of membrane receptors.

The dopamine hypersensitivity is shown schematically in the following figure. This should be compared to Figure 22 and 23 used earlier in the discussion of neuroleptic induced akinesia.

If the neuroleptic dose is decreased, the hypersensitivity response to dopamine increases because dopamine blockade is reduced. If the neuroleptic dose is increased, the symptoms of tardive dyskinesia decrease since the increased receptor blockade reduces hypersensitivity.

The drug producing the tardive dyskinesia can be used to "treat" the movement disorder and reduction of the drug makes the problem more apparent. Increasing the neuroleptic dose to prevent the symptoms of tardive dyskinesia only buys time before the problem recurs and requires a further

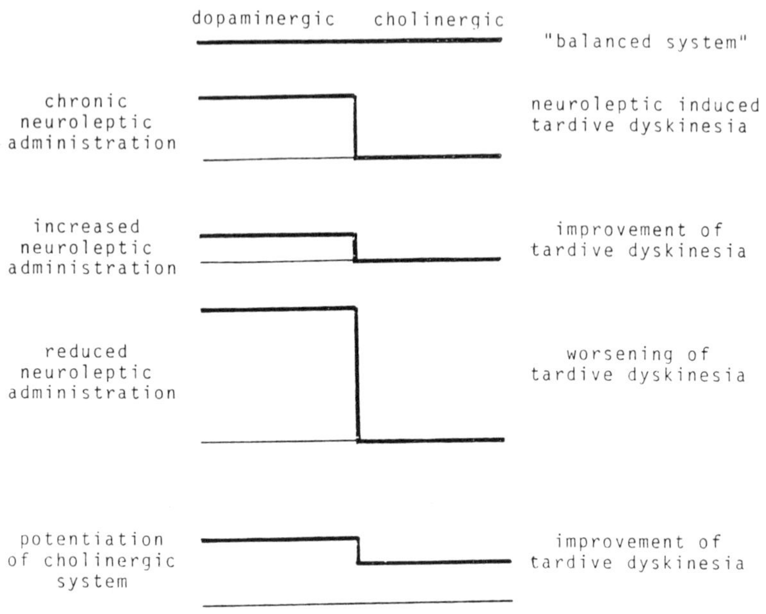

Figure 24

increase in neuroleptic dose. There is an upper limit of neuroleptics that can be given to the patient.

If the neuroleptic is discontinued or decreased, it is possible the patient will have a recurrence of his psychosis and/or worsening of the movement disorder may become intolerable. If, however, a small reduction in the neuroleptic dose is made there may be no significant change in the mental state and the worsening tardive dyskinesia may be tolerable. Over a period of months, the movement disorder may gradually improve as if the dopamine receptors are able to "repair" themselves. Patients on long term neuroleptic treatment should have periodic trials of reduction in drug dose. All patients should be given the minimum amount of medication which achieves the desired clinical effect.

Anticholinergic agents are not useful in treating tardive dyskinesia. Reference to Figure 24 shows that anticholinergic will "increase the imbalance" between the dopaminergic and cholinergic components. Perhaps the risk of developing tardive dyskinesia is increased if chronically treated patients received anticholinergics along with neuroleptics. This stresses the need to determine whether patients actually require anticholinergics for extrapyramidal side effects associated with neuroleptic therapy.

Use of anticholinesterases have been considered for treatment of tardive dyskinesia but their short duration of action in the central nervous system results in their failure for treatment of this syndrome.

The administration of choline to raise the cholinergic component is impractical. Administration of phosphatidylcholine (lecithin) which is an effective choline donor requires large amounts and the patient takes on an unpleasant fishy odor. The value of this treatment is not yet established.

Dopamine synthesis is controlled by an inhibitive feedback felt to be GABA mediated (Figure 22). The movement disorder of tardive dyskinesia may be treatable by giving GABA to decrease the synthesis of dopamine in the substantia nigra. This is the rationale for GABA in treatment of dyskinesia such as choreoathetosis. Neuroleptics can have same effect by blocking dopamine receptors in the corpus striatum.

12. Paradoxical Response

For some patients, the result of neuroleptic therapy is a worsening of the symptoms rather than an improvement. It is possible that more symptoms are elicitable because of improvement in such features as a formal thought disorder or lessening of a retarded catatonia.

The worsening of the clinical picture may be due to side effects of the neuroleptics such as akasthesia or sedation. This situation may require a change in neuroleptic. In rare cases, neuroleptics produce an acute organic brain syndrome with features of hyperthermia and autonomic nervous system dysfunction involving such as blood pressure and heart rate.

A worsening of the clinical picture should raise the possibility of an incorrect or incomplete diagnosis. There may be some unidentified toxic-organic factor contributing to the impaired mental state or the functional disorder is other than schizophrenia.

It must be stressed that if a patient's mental state improves with neuroleptics this does not prove that the patient was schizophrenic or that he suffered from a functional psychosis. At no point in this text have neuroleptics been called antischizophrenic agents. Also, the fact that a patient does not respond to a therapeutic trial of neuroleptics does not rule out schizophrenia. These agents are not a 'litmus test'' for schizophrenia.

CHAPTER 10

PSYCHOPATHOLOGY OF THE MAJOR AFFECTIVE DISORDERS

THE PSYCHOPATHOLOGY OF AFFECT

> Affect refers to a subjective and momentary emotional complex which often has physiological accompaniments. Mood is a feeling state which involves more prolonged and pervasive emotion.

Earlier in this text the major affective disorders were defined as

> A group of mental disorders characterised by symptoms which reflect problems in cognition, perception, affect, mobility and behaviour relating to a perturbation of affect. Usually a prominent feature of the mental state is a disturbance of mood.

The major affective disorders can be divided into *primary* and *secondary* disorders. The primary affective disorders are of functional etiology and their mental symptoms arise because of a core perturbation "located" in the affect component. The occurrence of symptoms ascribable to other components of the mental state indicates an extension of this perturbation within the composite mental state.

```
                  ┌ cognition
perturbation      ├ perception
     of          ─┤
   affect         ├ mobility
                  └ behaviour
```

Figure 25

The fact that a disturbed mental state has prominent or dominating affective symptoms does not automatically make for the diagnosis of a primary affective disorder. There are many other disorders, either of an organic or functional etiology, which can have a presentation dominated by affective symptomatology. These disorders constitute the secondary affective disorders. For instance, an adult adjustment disorder in response, for example, to the death of a spouse. A disorder of an organic etiology whose presentation can be dominated by affective symptoms is hypothyroidism.

In primary affective disorders, the cognition, perception, mobility and behaviour are invariably disturbed to some degree. It may be that at the time of presentation the symptoms arising from the perturbation of one of these components is more prominent than the affective symptoms. It does not follow that the dominant symptoms of a primary affective disorder are necessarily affective in nature.

In summary, not all disorders whose clinical presentation is dominated by affective symptoms are primary affective disorders and not all primary affective disorders have a clinical presentation dominated by affective symptoms. It is helpful to recall that not all patients presenting with chest pain have a myocardial infarction and not all myocardial infarctions feature chest pain as the dominant symptom.

Unless this point is recognised, then there is a great risk of making both false positive and false negative diagnoses of primary affective disorders. The symptom and the disorder are not synonymous. Unfortunately, affective terms such as depression and mania are frequently used interchangably to denote both symptoms and disorder and this leads to much confusion for both clinicians and patients.

Another factor adding to the diagnostic problem is that emotional complexes are personalized experiences. The form and content of both the verbal and non-verbal language used to communicate these experiences are idiosyncratic in the extreme. The resulting words, actions and gestures are ripe for misunderstanding, misinterpretation, miscommunication, and misdiagnosis.

To simplify a discussion of the *dysphoria* associated with the major affective disorders, the symptoms will be grouped under the headings of "*depression*" and "*mania.*"

1. "Depression"

This subjective dysphoria may be expressed by terms such as *depression, unhappy, sad, blue, gloomy, low, dejected, despondent, devastated* and so on. The mood may be further assessed as *blunted, flat, bland, unmodulated, unresponsive* and *barren.*

The affect is not totally impaired and pathological as a result of a major affective disorder. In general, normal sets of affective responses can exist despite severe impairment. The situation is similar to that discussed earlier in connection with the symptomatology of the schizophrenias.

In depression, the affect can be experienced and expressed symptomatically as *hostile, angry* and *irritable.* Invariable *anxiety* is present to a significant degree and in some cases may be the dominant affective symptom. Rather than being sustained, the mood may show *fluctuations* and notable *lability.* The point is that the affect and mood associated with depression need not be limited to gloom and retardation.

It is common for depressive symptoms to take on a physical colouring. This condition is *painful.* Perhaps the most common enquiry to assess a person's mood is "How do you feel?" The response often includes terms such as *hurt, aching, tired, fatigued* and *exhausted.*

In general, the other symptoms which may arise from the perturbed mental state are congruent with the affective symptoms. The fragmentation and incongruities between components of the mental state discussed earlier in connection with the schizophrenias is rarely seen in the major affective disorders. However, as will be discussed later, this is not always the case.

Classically, there is a *loss of self-esteem* associated with depression. Self-esteem refers to a feeling of the self as a whole being. This requires integrated ego functions with notions of identity, self-worth, integrity and role. A loss in self-esteem, indicating a perturbation of the mental state, is often reflected by feelings of *rejection, inferiority, self-blame, shame* and *guilt.*

The triad of *feelings of hopelessness, worthlessness* and *guilt* is classically linked to suicidal ideation. A downward spiral can occur involving all components of the mental state. The patient's situation becomes one of *interminable anguish* with them being unable to see a way out or an end to the turmoil.

Clinically, a depression can proceed to where the person's mental functioning becomes stagnant. The overall psychomotor presentation is akin to that found in some chronic organic brain syndromes. In fact the differentiation of such a retarded depression from an organic dementia is often very difficult. This distinction must be made since the former disorder is frequently reversible whilst the latter often is not.

2. "Mania"

The subjective emotional complex in mania may be reported as *cheerful, spirited, high, elated, euphoric* and so on. This sometimes results in comments such as "What's so bad about that?" Perhaps a better perspective of mania is achieved by recalling the word *maniac.*

A key feature of manic dysphoria is the *lability, impulsivity, explosivity* and *unpredictability* in mood regulation. Often, this quality is coupled with irritability and leads to a dysphoria which is best described as "nasty".

The mood has an *expansiveness* which reflects the lack of regulation and control. Sometimes, the elation is referred to as being "infectious" since it can strike an observer as witty and cute. However, because of the lability and disinhibitions of mania these euphorias can quickly take a "nasty" turn.

The words elation and euphoria should not be taken too literally since a sustained "serene state of grace" is a rare finding in mania. There is likely to be much *anxiety, anger* or *frustration* accompanying any elation and euphoria. This is fueled by the demanding nature of the symptoms and the frustrations which arise when the impulsive shifts are not instantly met and satisfied.

The elation and euphoria have an *oversensitivity* and *brittleness*. In part this reflects the instability of the mood and the accompanying anger and frustration. Many maniacs complain about the *tension* in mania. Perhaps they may "like it" for the moment or for short periods in the more subdued phase of the illness. Nevertheless, they are often painfully aware of the problems and difficulties associated with their condition particularly in its more severe forms.

The affect and mood seen in functional mania bears a striking similarity to that seen in some *frontal lobe syndromes*. This is an organic brain syndrome with causes such as trauma, tumors, and cerebrovascular accidents. Changes in the person's affect and behaviour are a feature of this syndrome. These changes are characterised by lability, suddenness and unpredictability. The affect can shift from a profound "depression" to a dramatic "mania" within the course of a single sen-tence. In some frontal lobe syndromes there is an incongruency between affect, cognition and behaviour. The precipitants which apparently trigger these swings are notably insignificant compared to the response which is aptly described as a *catastropic reaction*.

There is an increasing amount of clinical and neurophysiological evidence that inhibition is an important function of the frontal lobes. EEG analysis and positron emission tomography (PET) suggest abnormalities of the frontal areas of the brain in patients with functional mania. Perhaps some of the control and delaying of gratification outlined in the psychoanalytic theories reflect the development of the fronto-limbic system.

THE PSYCHOPATHOLOGY OF COGNITION

> Cognition is that operation of the mind by which one becomes aware of objects of thought and perception. It includes the processes of understanding and reason.

The model for cognition outlined in the discussion of the schizophrenias can be applied in this section. In the major affective disorders, the perturbation of cognition is due to an extension or invasion by the core disturbance from the affect component. It follows that any of the cognitive symptoms discussed earlier in connection with the schizophrenias can arise in the major affective disorders.

It is obvious that cognitive function will depend on the accompanying mood. To simplify a discussion of the cognitive symptoms associated with, though not pathognomonic of, the major affective disorders the symptoms will be grouped under the headings of "depression" and "mania."

1. "Depression"

The cognitive disturbance can produce a *formal thought disorder*. A person with significant depression will have difficulties *holding a cognitive set*. A frequent problem is a *loss in concentration*. There is a variant of the *interpenetration of themes* as depressive content contaminates the cognitive task at hand. The person's loss in concentration is because he cannot keep his mind on the job due to his thoughts wandering to depressive material. This symptom rarely takes the form of thought insertion of the type constituting a first rank symptom of schizophrenia although it is possible.

More often, the depressed person reports a *preoccupation* with depressive material. Cognitive function becomes more impaired when this preoccupation becomes a *rumination*. Here, there is an ongoing, non-productive internal debate involving the depressive material which can result in cognitive paralysis.

Frequently, this inability to concentrate is seen by the patient as a *memory impairment.* Psychological testing and the clinical interview may result in a picture identical to that seen in primary dementia. However, such a patient does not have dementia but rather a so-called *pseudodementia.* This word can be misleading since it has the suggestion of pretending or faking the deficit. It is better to refer to this feature as one of *reversible dementia* since in many cases treatment of the underlying depressive illness will alleviate the deficit.

The symptoms of reversible dementia due to a major affective disorder are of particular importance in geriatric patients. The possibility of a major depressive illness can be so easily overlooked in these patients. This is more likely if the patient has some "features" of chronic organic brain syndrome such as brain atrophy by CT scan.

Classically, the depressed patient displays *slowness* and *retardation* in thinking. There is a *poverty of thought and ideation* which is likely compounded by decreased concentration, preoccupations and ruminations. Once again, there is the danger of misdiagnoses such as organic dementia or mental retardation in many patients.

Rather than the cognitive feature being one of retardation, the picture may be dominated by apprehension, fear and dread. There is still an inability to hold a cognitive set but cognitive function is "agitated" by anxiety rather than retarded.

A patient with these cognitive difficulties can appear to be *confused* and *disoriented.* This consideration may arise because of his response and performance on psychological testing in addition to his observed behaviour. In depression, this is secondary rather than primary but it is important to consider an acute organic brain syndrome in the differential diagnosis.

As the depression develops, the patient will attempt to cope and deal with the situation. A probable first step will be an attempt to think of a cause, a reason or a precipitant for the dysphoria. This attempt will be made not only by the patient but by his friends and family. As was pointed out in connection with the schizophrenias, this maneuver is ripe for problems. These "precipitants" allow the person "understand" the depression and they may allow a means of coping with the situation. Frequently, what is identified as the problem is no such thing and focusing on it may make the situation worse. However, the lack of "cause" can lead to feelings of helplessness.

For instance, it may be concluded that the depression is due to the person losing his job. He or his associates can readily agree that this is "logical." This conclusion may be reinforced by recalling that "he only looked sad, unhappy and despondent after he got his severence letter." This could be the incorrect equating of the appearance of the depressive symptom with the onset of the depressive syndrome.

The loss of a job may be the result of a longstanding and unrecognised depression. The major, and unrecognised, symptoms could well have been an impaired concentration, poverty of ideation and preoccupation resulting in poor cognitive performance which culminated in the man's dismissal. If the man returns to work under these circumstances, without the underlying depressive illness being recognised and treated, then he is likely to fail once again. Each failure is a frustration and further loss of self-esteem and places another "Nail in the coffin."

Try as they may, patients at times fail to identify a cause for their depressive dysphoria. The search can become a preoccupation which further impairs their cognitive function. Notions of hopelessness, inadequacy, worthlessness and guilt are developed and amplified. The lack of a discernible reason for their depression means that they cannot "face" the problem and so cannot formulate any way out of the situation. The helplessness is further compounded by the fact that the cognitive functioning is becoming increasingly perturbed. The depressive begins to lose perspective from his family's point of view but the material is perfectly congruent and in perspective with his own thinking.

At times, the patients fabricate causes for their depressions which are both ridiculous and pathetic. For example, with total conviction, a patient may decide that "it's all due to my having cheated the government out of $250 on my income tax return in 1941." It is crucial to realise that this conviction is internally consistent with the patient's other cognitive sets and congruent with the other components which comprise his mental state.

Specific cognitive symptoms such as *paranoid ideation, overvalued ideas, misinterpretations, delusional perceptions* and *primary delusions* can arise in these disorders. The mechanisms for their development are the same as discussed earlier in connection with the schizophrenias. In the major affective disorders, there has been the necessary disturbance of cognition by the extension of the core perturbation from the affect component.

Specifically, the paranoid features of suspiciousness, hypervigilance and ideas of victimization may result from the person's impaired memory and concentration. He may feel that his employer is hostile when in fact he is being reasonably critical in view of the person's impaired work performance because of impaired concentration. The actions and interventions of the patient's family and friends can also be misinterpreted by the patient making the situation ripe for systematisation and secondary verification as the dysphoria progresses.

If the person's depressive illness is not recognised, then his associates may become critical and judgmental. This further adds fuel to the patient's ideas of victimisation and accelerates the downhill spiral. If the family is protective and tries to "ease the pressure on him," this may be interpreted by the patient as a snub or verification that he is inadequate and helpless. Delusional perceptions can arise via the "two-memberedness" discussed earlier in the text, leading to delusional ideas and pathologically derived convictions.

The type of primary delusion seen in depressive disorders is not restricted to being of a persecutory nature. Of particular interest are *dysmorphobic delusions*. These refer to the patient's body and may be such as the delusional conviction that the body is rotting and emitting a putrid odour. It is interesting that the patient often displays resignation, for example, that this rotting and putrid body is "just punishment for my transgressions and shows that I should be killed like the dog that I am."

These dysmorphobic features can be coupled with a *nihilistic* view of the world, illustrating the congruency between the components of the perturbed mental state. The world is viewed as "grey and colourless" and life as "as walking shadow, signifying nothing." This *anhedonic* fatalism and negation is seen in *Cotard's syndrome*, a subgroup of involutional melancholia, which is a type of major depressive syndrome.

2. "Mania"

The *formal thought disorder* seen in mania can result in any of the symptoms previously discussed in connection with the schizophrenias. There can be a *loosening of associations* and a *failure to hold a cognitive set* with *overinclusivity, interpenetration of themes, tangentiality* and *derailment.* In fact, these symptoms of thought disorder are often more florid in mania than in schizophrenia.

A feature of manic thought disorder is its *distractability.* Occurrences such as someone entering the room or the ringing of a telephone clearly become included in the manic's train of thought and cause a disruption. Since this overinclusivity and interpenetration is often linked to cues, an apparent "pattern" can be seen in the manic's shifting of cognitive sets. Rather than the incomprehensible and bizzare nature of the schizophrenic's thought disorder, there is an apparent *flight of ideas* in mania.

A version of Figure 4 can be drawn for mania. It represents a deficit in an "external filter" for environmental occurrences as well as the upset of the "internal filter" which was discussed in connection with the schizophrenias. This is shown schematically in the following figure.

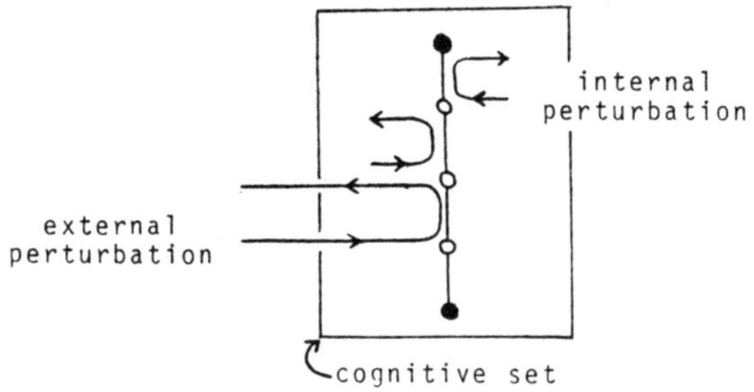

Figure 26

This external distractability and implosion by external stimuli results in a manic thought disorder which is *labile, fluctuating* and *variable*. This has many of the features seen in patients with toxic psychoses from street drugs or organic psychoses due to infection. The thought disorder of a manic placed in a quiet seclusion room is less florid than when he is on a busy ward. Reduction of external stimuli is an important feature in the clinical management of these patients. Nevertheless, even in seclusion, they display an "autonomous" lability.

Classically, the *rate of associations* is dramatically increased in mania due to the breakdown in filtering. There is a *pressure of speech* reflecting the implosion of cognitive material and failure to *contain* the cognitive set. The ability to communicate becomes impaired and the manic frequently becomes angry and frustrated by the apparent failure of others to "get the points being made." In some instances, the patient is well aware of the difficulties in expressing himself and reports that "My mouth cannot keep up with my mind." The speech can become garbled to the point of a word salad and lose its communicative value. The implosion of stimuli can become intense to the point of paralysing mental functioning and the manic "spins his wheels" in a mute catatonic state.

The manic's attention will be shortened and this is reflected by the shifting of topics and subsequent hyperactivity. The length of the attention span will determine the performance on digit span and serial 7 subtraction. For example, if the attention span is 20 seconds then the manic will correctly repeat a seven digit set in forward and reverse. Also, on serial sevens, he will be correct as far as the 60's and then will lose the set. This is in contrast to the patient with depression who will likely do poorly on the digit span and on the serial sevens from the outset.

The level of consciousness in mania will often appear to have a primary disturbance. The manic is likely to give indications of confusion and, perhaps, disorientation. However, mania does not have a primary alteration in the level of consciousness that is seen with acute organic brain syndromes. The confusion is a result of the disturbances in cognition due to the overall "implosion." Nevertheless, it is often difficult to differentiate mania from an acute drug toxic state.

Cognitive symptoms such as *paranoid ideation, ideas of reference, delusional perceptions* and *primary delusions* can arise in mania. As in the case of the schizophrenias, major depressive illness and toxic-organic psychoses there is a coexistence of pathological cognitive sets and non-pathological within the mental state. The cognitive symptoms which arise from the pathological sets are internally consistent with the non-pathological sets and as such are not "rejected" by the other components.

Classically, the delusions in mania are grandiose. An example would be a conviction, derived from a pathological cognitive set, that one has discovered perpetual motion. However, a sustained and purely grandiose delusion is somewhat rare since, understandably, the grandiose delusion quickly takes on a persecutory flavour. This may be secondary to the response and attitude of others to the declaration and to the individual's accounting for his failures and lack of recognition.

In female manics, the content of the grandiose primary delusion is often religious in nature. The delusion may begin as the conviction of being a second Virgin Mary but often developes features of persecution, for example, by the Protestants, Buddhists and Jews alike. In male manics, the grandiose content of the primary delusions is often business related. However, in many cases, this too develops a persecutory and litigious flavour.

Since this delusional material is usually coupled with congruent symptoms involving affect, perception, mobility and behaviour the manic is a formidable and difficult patient. The overall lability and disinhibition adds to the management problems and makes clinical intervention very difficult. As was mentioned earlier, mania is not a "desirable euphoria" nor can it be considered "fun" for either the patient or others. The delusional manics can cause havoc for himself and others which may never be repaired.

THE PSYCHOPATHOLOGY OF PERCEPTION

Perception is the conscious subjective awareness of objects and events in the environment (exteroception) and in one's body (interoception).

All of the symptoms arising from a distortion of perception in the schizophrenias can occur in major affective disorders. As in the schizophrenias, the pathological and non-pathological perceptual sets coexist in the mental state. The nature of the perceptual symptoms in the major affective disorders depends on the degree of "invasion" by the affect perturbation into the perception component. In general, the responses from the other components which comprise the mental state are congruent with the perceptual phenomena.

1. "Depression"

Symptoms include *misperception, illusions* and *hallucinations.* These can take a variety of forms such as auditory, visual, olfactory and somatic.

The content of these symptoms usually potentiate the loss of self-esteem, guilt, hopelessness and despondency of the depression. They variously accuse, condemn, ridicule and criticise the patient.

The olfactory hallucinations may comprise offensive odours which add to the patient's gloom and "help to explain" why he is shunned and avoided by colleagues. The somatic hallucinations can have dysmorphobic features, for instance, the patient may report "feeling" a cancer spreading inside his brain. In Cotard's syndrome, a patient may smell, feel and see the effects of the delusional decomposition of his body. The world is not only reasoned as being grey and colourless but is perceived by the senses as such in this state of *negation.*

2. "Mania"

A characteristic of the perception is its *distractability.* This influences the patient's mental state in more components than perception. The perceptual difficulties reflect in, for example, impulsive and erratic behaviour as the patient fails to adequately "filter out" environmental stimuli.

The perception component of the mental state is *assaulted, flooded, imploded* and *overloaded* by all manner of stimuli. The break-down of the "external filter" means a failure to delay, organise and reject stimuli. In some cases, the patients are driven to the point of distraction and exhaustion because of this state of *hypersensitivity* and can become confused and disoriented to the point of "delirium." In manics with a significant degree of perceptual disturbance, the differentiation from an acute organic brain syndrome is particularly difficult. As in the case of the depressive syndrome, these perceptual symptoms tend to compound the manic state. The distraction particularly increases the cognitive and behavioural difficulties.

THE PSYCHOPATHOLOGY OF MOBILITY

> Mobility refers to the mental representation of will, drive and volition which initiates voluntary speech and movement.

As pointed out earlier, catatonia has more than one possible etiology. It can be due to toxic organic factors, schizophrenia or a major affective disorder. The symptoms of mobility discussed in connection with the schizophrenias can be found in major affective disorders. The viewpoint that agitated and retarded catatonia may reflect phenomena such as passivity of volition, response to hallucinations and compliance with primary delusions applies equally to the major affective disorders as it does to the schizophrenias.

1. "Depression"

The most common finding is a decrease in the patient's mobility. This is often referred to by the patient as weakness, fatigue or lack of initiative. This *retarded catatonia* can progress to the point of anergia and can develop secondary life-threatening features. The patient's speech reflects an accompanying cognitive problem akin to the motor impairment which can result in mutism. He cannot formulate mentally the notion for initiation of voluntary actions let alone carry them out.

In depression, the mobility may be *agitated* and *hyperactive* rather than hypomobile. It should be stressed that not all depressive syndromes feature motor retardation. If anxiety is a prominent symptom and the patient experiences "painful" cognitive and perceptual symptoms, then the motor presentation may be one of *restlessness* and *agitated pacing.* This *agitated catatonia* is a feature of the depressive syndrome of involutional melancholia.

2. "Mania"

Agitated mobility is a feature of mania. The *verbal and motor stereotypies* discussed in schizophrenia can occur in this major affective disorder. The overactivity may drive the patient to physical and mental exhaustion which can have serious sequelae.

This driven quality may have the features of *passivity.* The manic feels compelled to overactivity and complain of his inability to oppose these urges. It is possible that the agitation becomes disorganised to a degree resulting in *hypomobility.* He is "spinning his wheels" to the point of inaction.

THE PSYCHOPATHOLOGY OF BEHAVIOUR

Behaviour is defined as all those observable actions which establish and influence interpersonal relationships and have a major influence on the lifestyle.

Clearly, behaviour is significantly altered by the major affective disorders. In turn, the resulting interactions with others will alter the clinical features of the major affective disorders. An initial assessment of an individual's personality, frequently based on his mood and behaviour, should not be, but often is, taken at face value in diagnosing a major affective disorder.

1. "Depression"

The usual behaviour associated with depression can be summarized as a *withdrawal.* This indicates a retardation in the person's mental and physical functioning and may also reflect the person's loss of self-esteem and inability to cope.

The withdrawal may go unrecognised for a long period of time if it is not inconvenient or disruptive to others. If the person's mood is not obviously sad and unhappy, then the likelihood of overlooking a major depressive disorder as the etiology of withdrawal is particularly increased. Indeed, under these circumstances, the withdrawal may result in criticism of the individual and the conclusion that he is cold and "not worth the bother."

The ultimate withdrawal is *suicide.* The most common type, *egoistic,* is characterised by the person perceiving a lack of support systems with the interminable anguish experienced in social isolation. Usually, there is a gradual buildup of suicidal ideation based on both pathological and non-pathological mental sets and this congruent blend finally reaches a critical level. It is important to realise that the "lethal level" is not necessarily maintained all of the time. As in the brief reactive psychoses, there is a fluctuation in the stresses around a "flash point." A major affective disorder can be a potent catalyst in peaking into the critical state. However, it must be strongly emphasised that suicide does not necessarily mean that the person has a major affective disorder.

A common myth regarding suicide is that those who "back out" were not serious in their intent. One example is the overdose patient who then calls an ambulance to take them to a hospital. In a perjorative way, it is often concluded that he was manipulative and only seeking attention by a gesture. However, it may be that the person had concluded in desperation that only hospitalisation would get the required attention. Many of the "ambulance callers" are "proctalgic" manipulators but this is by no means always the case. Perhaps the myth is continued by clinicians to give them a concrete "fact" to lessen their own anxiety and sense of helplessness when faced with suicide cases.

Probably, for a limited period, the person "really wants to die" since the multiple factors have reached a critical level. However, swallowing pills or slashing a blood vessel is not an instantaneous death and allows for a period of reflection, doubt and panic which can result in a change of mind.

For many, the overdose starts out as simply "wanting to go to sleep for a long time" with the hope that when they awake the "problems will be over." Often, the sleeping pills lead to a drowsy state and the number of pills taken is miscalculated. It is said that as many as 40 percent of barbiturate overdoses are "mistakes" due to a drug induced confusion with an automation-like taking of more barbiturates.

As part of the overall withdrawal, detachment and behavioural isolation, a depressed patient may show aggressive, and agitated behaviour. He becomes quarrelsome, mercurial and self-destructive which speeds his rejection and abandonment. Suicide is a hostile act which is not only directed against the self but also toward others. There is a clear expression of anger towards those who remain alive with the notion that they may have "failed" the suicide in some way. Many suicidal patients display *inimcability* in that their actions make them their own worse enemies. They block, oppose and resist attempts to offer support and assistance.

Abuse of alcohol, "uppers" and "downers" are a common behavioural feature in depression. Initially, these substances may relieve the dysphoria by "brightening" the patient or, on the other hand, "numbing" his awareness of the problems for a time. In some cases, being able to "cry in his beer" may help the patient organize and express some of the problems which can be beneficial. However, these "benefits" are quickly lost and the continued substance abuse begins to add its own problems to the clinical picture. It is often difficult to decide whether substance abuse is a primary or secondary feature in major depressive disorders.

2. "Mania"

The behavioural changes associated with depression may go unnoticed for a considerable length of time, but this is unlikely to be the case in mania. The labile, distractable and disinhibited quality of manic symptoms quickly results in attention.

The formal thought disorder with flight of ideas and pressure of speech does not facilitate the manic "fading into the background." Similarly other cognitive symptoms and symptoms relating to affect, perception and mobility do not lend themselves to behavioural disguise. The *demanding* nature of the symptoms, the *lack of judgement,* and *impulsivity* produce a disruptive lifestyle for both the patient and his associates which soon reaches pathological proportions.

During the early phase of mania, or in its mild version, the patient may experience "life in the fast lane" as both desirable and productive. He presents a "hail fellow well met" quality and it is said that such manics make excellent "travelling salesmen." Obviously, attempts at clinical intervention are met with resistance from the manic. The patient finds the circumstances and situation to be congruent with his mental status and shows little or no insight as regards any problems. It is unfortunate that much damage can be caused during this phase for the patient and his family. In many instances, this damage cannot be repaired when the mania has been resolved.

In severe mania, the patient is often far from "comfortable" with his circumstances. The lack of constraints frequently puts him at odds with society. It should be noted that it is not the "deviant and troublesome" behaviour which makes for the diagnosis of psychopathology but rather the pathological processes which result in these problems. For example, it is not the fact that manics "go on irresponsible spending sprees" that is pathological but rather the cognitive, affective, perceptual and mobility dysfunctions resulting in this behaviour which constitutes the mental disorder.

It is more likely that substance abuse will arise during mania than during depression. The manic state lends itself to "frequenting bars more than libraries." Alcohol and drugs will reduce whatever constraints are still present in mania.

Primary suicidal ideation based on a loss of self-esteem is not a feature of mania. Nevertheless, mania has a notable morbidity and lethality since the disinhibited behaviour can certainly put the person at physical risk.

The functional psychoses have a "malignancy" in the sense that they are not experienced in isolation but rather impinge on the functioning of others. A parent operating from a depressed position can have significantly detrimental effects on the development of their children particularly during early childhood. The behavioural influences of a manic on his family and associates is particularly "malignant." From the patient's developmental viewpoint, the establishment and maintenance of meaningful interpersonal relationships is impaired even in mild cases of mania. The development of a "healthy" personality and outlook is also likely to be impaired.

CHAPTER 11

DIAGNOSTIC CONSIDERATIONS IN MAJOR AFFECTIVE DISORDERS

This is far from being a simple topic. The major affective disorders do not have exclusive or pathognomonic symptoms. The presence of a dysphoric *symptom* does not necessarily imply the existence of a major affective disorder. The major affective disorders need not feature the layman's notion of "obvious" symptoms. For example, a major depressive disorder need not have its clinical presentation dominated by sadness. Furthermore, many of the associated symptoms can occur from a "normal response" to life stress and it is critical to identify such cases before prescribing treatment.

From a clinical viewpoint, the major affective disorders post a distinct "chicken or egg" problem. As an example, consider a patient who has a cancer with poor prognosis who is recognised as becoming "severely depressed" during the chemotherapy. There are a number of formulations regarding the person's mental state: 1) the depression is "natural and understandable"; 2) the patient has a major affective disorder which is simply compounded and amplified by the cancer problem; 3) the patient has a major affective disorder and the cancer problem adds little to the overall condition; 4) the "severe depression" is an organic disorder due to the cancer and the side effects of chemotherapy; 5) the patient's problem is a major depressive disorder complicated by the psycho-social problems of the cancer plus the toxic-organic problems of the cancer and the chemotherapy. All one has to do is sort out the "etiology."! The first step is to recognise, and not be defeated by, the fact that this is not a simple problem. The information that the patient "did not appear depressed until told of his cancer" does not necessarily clarify the situation though many clinicians would be sorely tempted to draw a conclusion.

The diagnostic classification of major affective disorders is best approached from biological, psychological and sociological viewpoints. This approach is probably more necessary than in the case of the schizophrenias because of the very nature of affective illness.

The following discussion of diagnostic features of the major affective disorders reflects the zeitgeist. As one reviews some of the diagnostic classifications their biases, which in many instances are reflections of the available "technology," are apparent.

KRAEPELIN

The functional psychoses were divided by Kraepelin into *dementia praecox* and *manic depressive disorders.* He paid particular attention to the natural course of these two disorders in their delineation. The manic-depressive disorders differed from dementia praecox in that they had a course characterised by remissions and relapses. During the remission period, the manic-depressive patient returned to his premorbid level of functioning. The progressive deterioration of dementia praecox was not seen in manic-depressive disorders.

The manic-depressive episode was either of a depressed or a manic type. For some patients, all episodes were a depressed phase. For others, both manic and depressed phases occurred in the course of the disorder. A frequently used schematic representation of the manic-depressive disorder is a sinusoidal curve depicting a cycling of "highs" and "lows" with a fixed periodicity. This is a rare clinical finding. The more likely representation is shown in the following figure.

Often, the manic and depressive episodes occur in groups rather than alternating and do not repeat at fixed intervals.

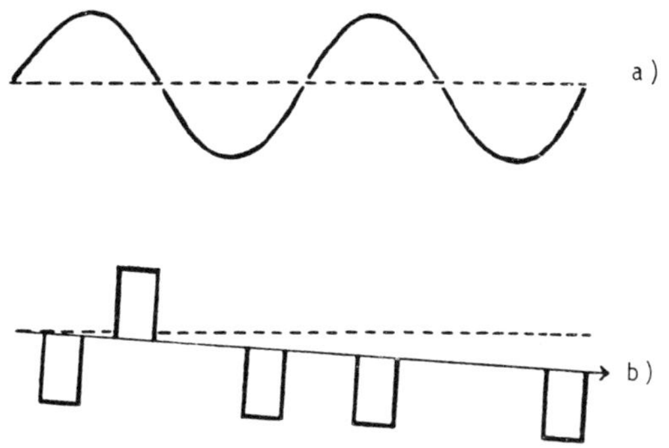

Figure 27

As would be expected with any severe clinical disorder, there is some degree of impairment in the patient's overall level of functioning over a chronic course. Despite the alleviation of an episodes' symptoms there is likely to be some secondary residual deficiency.

SYMPTOM CLUSTERING

There is a wide range of symptoms associated with the major affective disorders. If certain symptoms group or cluster together in their clinical presentation, then this could provide a means of classifying the disorders.

Some studies suggested that this clustering of symptoms occurred. The clustering of the more common symptoms was bimodal with a distinct boundary between the two symptom groupings. The result was a diagnostic splitting of the major depressive disorders into two types. This is schematically shown in the following figure.

The *biological* versus *psychological* classification of depressive syndromes reflects the "nature versus nurture" approach. The biological symptom cluster has also been referred to as *vegetative* and *endogenous*. Many of the symp-

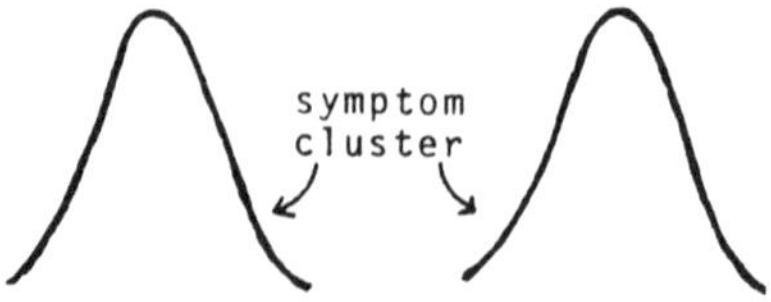

biological endogenous vegetative	psychological exogenous reactive
psychotic	neurotic
(primary)	(secondary)

Figure 28

toms in this cluster are expressed in physiological terms, for instance, sleep disturbance, loss of appetite and decreased weight. The vegetative aspects include loss of energy, withdrawal and loss of initiative and drive. The depressive syndrome characterised by these biological and vegetative symptoms tend to run a relatively autonomous course which is not particularly influenced by external factors. The symptoms display an endogenous rather than exogenous or reactive quality.

The psychological symptom cluster does not include the symptoms of the biological clustering. Its symptoms show a *reactive* nature, for example, responses to external stresses such as job pressure, marital strife and social conflicts are featured. An exogenous rather than autonomous quality is seen in the symptoms and their course. However, this reactivity point could be misleading if it is taken to mean that the biological or endogenous depressions symptoms do not have a responsivity to external events.

Psychotic symptoms such as hallucinations and delusions can occur in major depressive disorders. A division of depression into *psychotic* and *neurotic* can be made depending on whether or not such symptoms occur. It is more likely that psychotic symptoms will be associated with the biological depressions. The neurotic subclassification of depression is misleading because the term neurotic is now generally used in a judgmental and prejorative sense to imply that the patient simply needs to display some "intestinal fortitude." In this sense, it "belittles" the seriousness of the condition.

The biomodal clustering of symptoms has implications in terms of the appropriate treatment for the two depressive disorders. The biological or endogenous depression featuring vegetative symptoms is more likely to respond to somatic treatments such as psychopharmacology. The psychological or reactive type depression is likely to require psycho-social intervention rather than medications and the effectiveness of the latter is likely to be minimal.

However, in clinical practice, in "reality," a clear-cut bimodal clustering of depressive symptoms is rarely the case. The previous figure is more correctly drawn in the following manner.

There is an overlap in the symptom groupings rather than a distinct split with a combination of biological, psychological and sociological features. In a sense, one has to "place" a given patient at some point on the horizontal

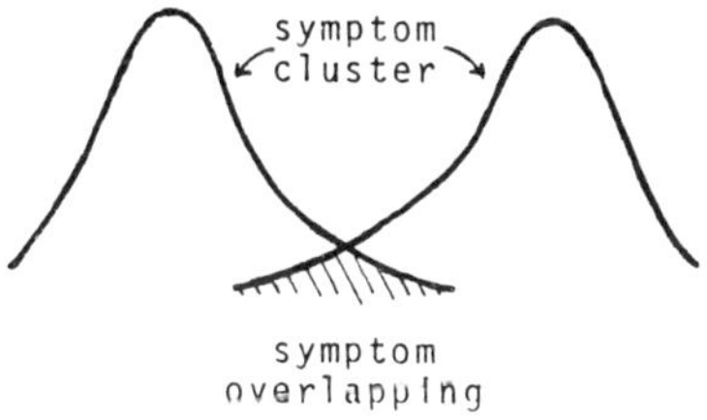

biological endogenous vegetative	psychological exogenous reactive
psychotic	neurotic
(primary)	(secondary)

Figure 29

axis depending on the particular mixture of symptoms. This placement returns to the notion mentioned earlier in the text of *primary* versus *secondary* depressive disorders.

The ability to correctly choose the treatment modalities is crucial. This is particularly the case given the effectiveness of modern psychopharmacology. However, it would be naive to think that a medication would significantly influence depressive symptoms arising from, say, an acute financial crisis.

It is a gross oversimplification to imply that such complex and diverse conditions as the major affective disorders can be classified neatly into two exclusive groups. Nevertheless, this approach is clinically helpful if its limitations are borne in mind. The symptoms which show a clustering tendency will be discussed in detail later in this chapter.

PRIMARY AND SECONDARY AFFECTIVE DISORDERS

By definition, the primary affective disorders are of functional etiology. The symptom profile arises from a core disturbance located in the affect component of the mental state. Patients must have no past history or current indications of disorders such as schizophrenia, neuroses, personality disorders or adjustment reactions which could account for the presenting symptom profile. In addition, there must be no past or present indication of toxic-organic disorders, such as endocrinopathies, drug therapy or substance abuse which could account for the patient's symptomatology.

The primary affective disorders are a diagnosis of strict exclusion. The inability to exclude these other factors, for instance a strong history of substance abuse or previous schizophrenic episodes necessitates a diagnosis of a *secondary affective disorder* for the current presentation. This is schematically shown in the following figure.

It has been stressed throughout this text that there are no pathognominic symptoms differentiating the functional from the toxic-organic psychoses. In addition, there are no symptoms which exclusively separate the schizophrenias

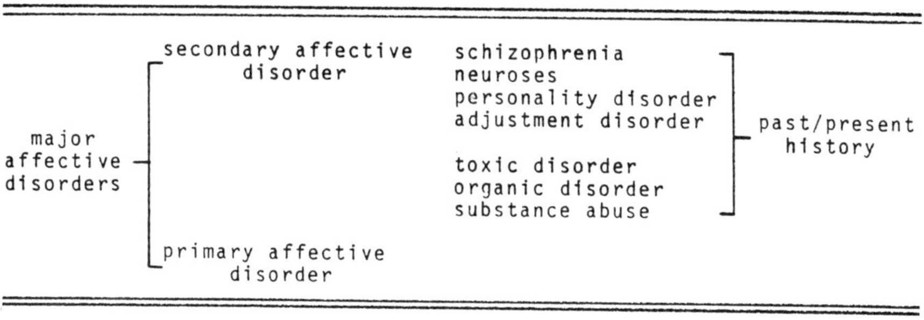

Figure 30

from the major affective disorders. Furthermore, it follows that no symptom differentiates the primary from the secondary affective disorders.

The schizophrenias can have a clinical presentation which is dominated by affective symptoms. Furthermore, the schizophrenias can have prominent symptoms such as impaired concentration, sleep disturbance and decreased appetite, which can be characteristic of major depressive illness. It is necessary to work through a differential diagnosis. The need to differentiate a primary depressive disorder from a secondary depressive disorder is crucial. The first will likely respond to antidepressants as the major form of therapy whilst the latter would require fundamentally different types of treatment.

Hypothyroidism can alter brain function and result in symptoms such as impaired concentration, sleep disturbance, decreased appetite as well as profoundly depressed facies. It must be realised that these mental symptoms can present long before this endocrinopathy produces signs such as dry skin, hoarse voice, decreased deep tendon reflexes or loss of the outer third of the eyebrow.

A patient who presents with these mental symptoms without the classical physical findings, so-called "masked myxoedema," is very likely to be misdiagnosed as having a primary depressive illness. If antidepressants are then prescribed, not only will they fail to alleviate the mental symptoms but may well prove dangerous in such a hypometabolic state. The mental symptoms in this case could probably be relieved with the use of thyroid hormone.

The primary versus secondary affective disorder diagnostic division has a particular advantage, namely, that it forces the clinician to work through a comprehensive differential diagnosis. This approach stresses and reinforces that there is a commonality of symptoms for toxic-organic psychoses, the schizophrenias and the major affective disorders as well as for a number of other psychiatric disorders.

The consideration, investigation, ruling out and, if necessary, the treatment of these other functional and toxic-organic disorders, some of which are given in Figure 30, illustrates the psychiatrist's role. These disorders cannot be dealt with or ruled out unless the clinician is aware of their signs and symptoms and considers them. Perhaps one could define a psychiatrist as a physician who is aware of the implications of, and pays attention to, changes in a patient's mental state of both functional and toxic-organic etiologies.

BIPOLAR AND UNIPOLAR DISORDERS

The primary affective disorders can be divided into *bipolar* and *unipolar disorders* as shown in the following figure.

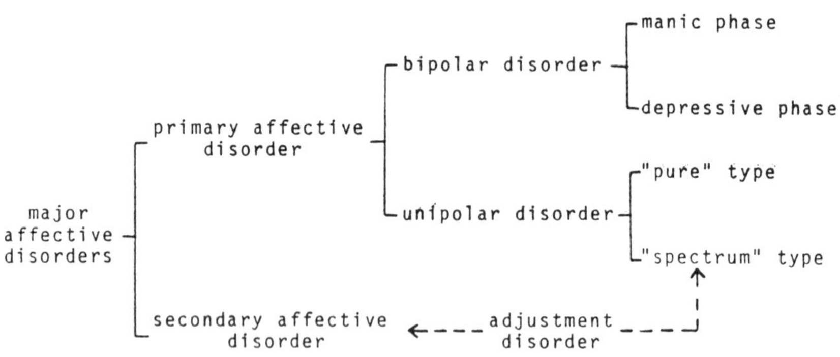

Figure 31

If all episodes occurring in the course of a primary affective disorder are of the depressive phase, then, by definition, this is a unipolar disorder. If in the course of a primary depressive disorder a manic phase occurs, then, by definition, this is a bipolar disorder. These points are schematically shown in the following figure.

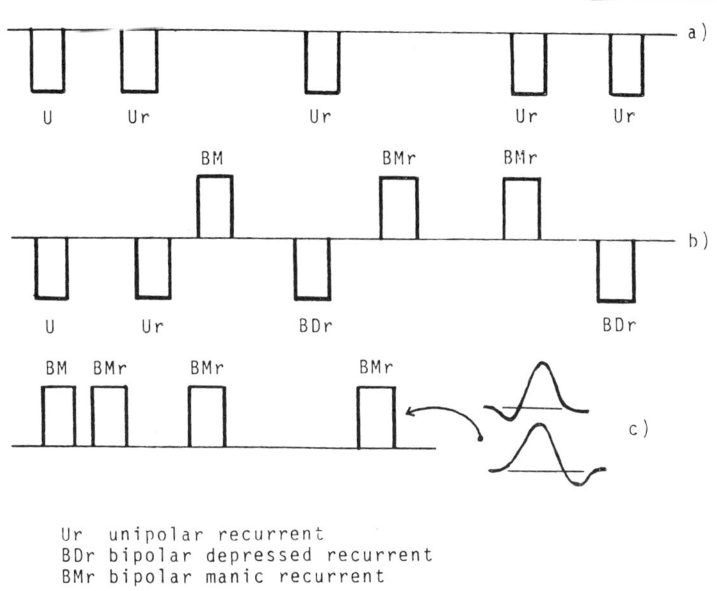

Figure 32

It is the occurrence of a manic episode at some point in the natural course of a primary affective disorder which defines the bipolar disorder. The bipolar disorder is not defined in terms of alternating depressed and manic episodes. Some 10 to 20 percent of patients with bipolar disorders have their first three episodes of the depressive type. The later occurrence of a manic episode requires a reclassification of what had been considered to be a unipolar disorder to bipolar disorder. This point is illustrated in the preceding figure.

Primary affective disorders featuring recurrent manic episodes without depressive phases in the course of the illness are classified as bipolar. This pure recurring mania is a rare condition. If manic episodes are looked at in detail, it is apparent that they are invariably triphasic in nature as illustrated in the previous figure. The manic episode which quickly results in hospitalisation often has a preceeding depressive component which goes unrecognised. Similarly, the manic phase followed by a depressive component often has the depressive part overlooked in comparison to the mania, in fact the depression may be taken as a sign of improvement when in point it is pathological.

It must be borne in mind that treatment of either phase of a bipolar disorder risks the precipitation of the other phase. This stresses the need for careful observation during hospitalisation and outpatient followup. The manic patient may slip into a depressed phase a few weeks after discharge with suicidal complications and the previously bipolar depressive receiving antidepressant may go "high" a number of weeks after discharge.

There are other factors which differentiate the bipolar and unipolar primary affective disorders. On the average, the bipolar disorders begin their presentation some 15 years earlier than the unipolar. This is particularly the case in males. The untreated episodes of the bipolar disorder are generally of shorter duration than the unipolar. Typically, the untreated bipolar episodes run three to six months whereas the unipolar depressions have an average untreated duration of six to nine months. Approximately half of the unipolar patients only have a single episode and relapses are more common in the bipolar than unipolar disorders.

A positive family history of major depressive disorders is common in both bipolar and unipolar patients. The first degree relatives of bipolar patients tend to have bipolar illnesses, and those of unipolar patients, illnesses of the unipolar type. In general, a positive family history is more likely to be found in bipolar patients. This may be due in part to symptoms of mania in a relative being more likely "remembered" by the family than symptoms of depression. Also, alcoholism and substance abuse is more common in mania than in depression and can produce long remembered social disruption.

There is no consistent difference in the symptoms seen in the depressive phase of the bipolar and unipolar disorders. This emphasises the point that bipolar disorders may appear in the first few episodes to be unipolar in nature. The depressive symptoms of the bipolar and unipolar disorders will essentially respond equally to pharmaco-therapy and convulsive treatments (ECT). However, the "antidepressant" effect of lithium may be better in the bipolar disorders than in the unipolar. This point will be discussed later in the text.

As shown in Figure 31, the unipolar disorder can be further divided into *pure* and *spectrum disorders.* This division is based on a number of clinical factors. The pure unipolar disorder has its onset after the age of forty and is equally present in males and females. The incidence of psychiatric disorders in the relatives of these patients is not strikingly different from that of the general population. However, if there is a positive family history for psychiatric disorders, it tends to be of a depressive illness.

The spectrum unipolar disorder generally presents prior to forty years of age and is much more common in females. There is a notably high incidence of general psychiatric disorders in the first degree relatives of these patients. The female relatives tend to have disorders of a depressive nature which fall into the secondary affective disorder group rather than the primary. The male relatives of spectrum unipolar patients have a high incidence of sociopathy and alcoholism.

The spectrum unipolar patients can present with so-called biological and vegetative symptoms, but there is a strong overlay of marital, social and economic problems. It was said earlier in this chapter with reference to Figure 29 that there is an overlapping of symptom clusters and a major clinical task was "placing" a given patient on the horizontal axis. This problem presents in terms of the spectrum unipolar patients. The broken line in Figure 31 represents an axis similar to that in Figure 29 which "links" the primary affective disorders to the secondary type through the spectrum unipolar disorder.

This "placement" of a given patient is a practical issue in determining the relative need for biological, psychological and sociological interventions in the overall treatment. The total picture of a case raises such questions as "Does this case warrant a therapeutic trial of antidepressants or would a social worker be more appropriate?" or "Are we dealing with a depression that would respond better with a psychosocial approach as the main treatment modality and would medications be of any value?" The need for antidepressants "decreases" as one "moves" to the spectrum unipolar disorder and across to the secondary affective disorder due to, for example, an acute situational disturbance because of failed university examinations.

The "purest" of primary affective disorders will result in secondary psychological and sociological symptoms. Therefore, the dichotomy problem will always be present to some degree and there will always be the need for a *triple* approach to treatment involving biological, psychological and sociological modalities.

The remainder of this chapter is concerned with the *descriptive aspects* of the symptoms characteristic of the primary affective disorders. They are given in a somewhat "checklist" format. It should be recalled that the number of symptoms elicited from a given patient and the ones that dominate the clinical presentation may vary over time.

DESCRIPTIVE ASPECTS OF PRIMARY DEPRESSION

The following subheadings are not listed in order of importance or frequency. In a particular patient, some symptoms may not be present and the dominant symptoms vary from patient to patient. Clearly, the manner in which the particular symptom is communicated will vary from patient to patient. However, the *form* of the symptoms is the same which makes for a more objective and less interpretive approach to the diagnosis and allows for this descriptive discussion.

1. Alteration in Sleep

A depression related change in the sleep pattern may involve an increase, though more likely a decrease, in the patient's total sleep time. The sleep is characterised by frequent awakenings and the fact that, subjectively, the patient does not feel rested after sleeping. This feeling of being unrested is the case whether the sleep time has become prolonged or shortened.

Classically, in primary depression, there is *terminal insomnia,* which is characterised by an abrupt awakening in the early morning hours. The patient has difficulty going back to sleep resulting in his pacing the floor or lying in bed staring at the ceiling.

The use of hypnotics may result in the patient being "unconscious for eight hours" and the night nurse reporting that the patient slept through the night. Nevertheless, the patient will report that he is not rested and may insist that he did not sleep despite what the nurse reports. The point of dispute is not the quantity as much as it is the quality of sleep.

Rather than, or in addition to, terminal insomnia the patient may show *initial insomnia.* Upon retiring, the patient has problems falling asleep. There is much tossing and turning and during this time the patient may be preoccupied with "depressing" issues. These issues are likely to increase as the person becomes more fatigued due to the continuing sleep disturbance.

In the "light" sleep associated with periods of both initial and terminal insomnia as well as the multiple awakenings throughout the night, there is the likelihood of hypnogogic and hypnopompic hallucinations. The occurrence of these symptoms will compound the patient's depressive state.

The sleep EEG recording in these patients invariably shows a disruption from the normal pattern. The REM stages can be altered such that they become progressively shorter as the night wears on rather than the normal situation of a progressive prolongation. Studies show a tendency for the REM-latency, the time lapse between the onset of sleep and the occurrence of the first REM episode, to decrease in primary depressive disorders.

A significant percentage of the night's slow wave sleep Stage 4 normally occurs during the REM-latency period. This is an important stage of sleep, so much so that it is often referred to as restitutive sleep. In cases of primary depression with decreased REM-latency, there is a significant loss of Stage 4 sleep.

As the patient recovers from the depression, it is noted that there is a reverting of the sleep EEG patterns to normal. The REM-latency period becomes prolonged with a recovery of Stage 4 sleep and restoration of the REM phases occurs. There is a loss of Stage 4 sleep associated with normal aging and it is seen in schizophrenics but neither shows the progressive restoration features seen in many of the recovering primary depressive patients.

These alterations in the sleep EEG recordings are not found in all primary depressive cases. However, these changes do have clinical value and interesting theoretical implications. For example, a prolongation of REM-latency and increased Stage 4 sleep is reported to occur within a few days of beginning treatment with tricyclic antidepressants. These EEG changes may occur before notable alterations in the clinical symptoms are seen and suggest that such changes could be an important early indicator of the medication's therapeutic effect. It is often said that the patient's subjective improvement in the quality of his sleep is an early clinical finding as the depressive syndrome improves.

The fact that in many cases general hypnotics fail to produce a beneficial sleep whilst tricyclic antidepressants do is intriguing. Perhaps this points to the sleep disorder as a direct product of the underlying endogenous depression. However, this does not mean that antidepressants are necessarily better than hypnotics for patients with sleep disturbances which are unrelated to a primary depressive illness. Antidepressants are not generally indicated, for example, in patients with postoperative stress or acute life stress who complain of insomnia. The later may well be the most common cause of sleep disruption. It must be remembered that antidepressants are not without side effects and as little as one and a half grams is a lethal overdose for most people.

2. Alteration in Appetite

A depression related change in appetite may involve an increase but more typically it is a loss of appetite. Although there is often an accompanying alteration in weight which can be quantified or estimated, it is the appetite change that is the significant point.

This symptom of reduced appetite may be expressed as a decreased interest or enjoyment of food due to its bland taste or lack of appetizing smell. There is a loss of pleasure associated with eating and it becomes a chore.

It is important to differentiate between appetite and eating. For example, a housewife suffering from a primary depression may still cook meals and eat them with her family due to social pressure rather than being motivated by appetite. A patient may say that a weight loss is due to dieting but on further questioning may comment that, unlike in the past, the diet has been easier to carry through. In these two examples, appetite has been primarily impaired though only one patient had a loss of weight.

In a major depressive disorder, the patient may not eat because of feelings of worthlessness and guilt making him unworthy. In cases of primary depression, featuring paranoid ideation or persecutory delusions he may conclude that the food has been tampered with and could be harmful. The symptom of retarded catatonia in a depressive illness may result in the person being unable to feed himself.

If the appetite loss is a symptom of a primary depressive disorder, then it will likely improve with treatment of the depression. This does not mean that antidepressants are primary appetite stimulants.

Although a decrease is the most common change in appetite associated with depressive illness it is possible that the change may involve an increase in appetite. As in the case of the sleep disturbance, the change in the parameter is probably more important than the direction.

3. Diurnal Variation

The patient may describe a subjective variation in his overall mood and general sense of well-being during the day which is more than a simple reflection of encountered stresses. Classically, in primary depressive disorders the mood is at its worst and most debilitating in the early part of the day. The patient awakens "with a black cloud hanging over him" and an anergic dread of the coming day's tasks.

Throughout the day, much the result of functioning from a depressed state, the patient encounters stresses and difficulties which add to his dysphoria. It is striking that despite this accumulation of incidents he retrospectively concludes that his overall mood was at its "lowest" in the mornings.

This diurnal variation, at its worst in the early part of the day, strikes many of the patients as somewhat paradoxical. The inference is that the basic mood is "internally" defined and the daily stress is a perturbation on this endogenously determined state. The mood has an "autononomous" quality and as such may lead patients to feelings of futility as regards what they can do to alter their dysphoria.

The "autonomous" quality of the mood variation leads to the question of the role of precipitants in primary depressive disorders. Clearly, in any medical disorder, stress factors arise and contribute to the clinical picture but the crucial issue is to place them in perspective.

4. Precipitants

The role of precipitants in major functional disorders was mentioned earlier in connection with the schizophreniform psychoses. The question of precipitants and stress factors as a necessary and sufficient factor in major depressive disorders is an even more complex issue.

It is natural for the patient, his relatives and physicians to search for plausible precipitants of the depressive episode. Precipitants will provide a focus to help comprehend and deal with the problem. If there is no discernable "reason or cause" for the illness then the patient cannot organise a plan to combat the feelings and this amplifies the helplessness and hopelessness of the depression.

However, so-called precipitants can be dangerous and misleading. They may simply be incorrect and not causative facts or be given too much "weight." There is a tendency to take precipitant identification to imply that one "understands" the patient's disorder which may be comforting for all concerned but it could be tragically incorrect. For example, a medical student whose sadness, dejection and suicidal ideation became apparent after he failed his examinations could have been suffering from an unrecognised primary depression for many months. The examination failure may have been a result of this unrecognised depressive illness rather than its cause. Earlier symptoms such as difficulties concentrating, loss of energy, disruption of sleep pattern and decreased appetite with weight loss may have gone unrecognised or were "written off" as normal for a student with upcoming examinations. The depressive disorder did not necessarily start with the appearance of sadness and despondency since after all the disorder and the symptom are not synonymous.

Classically, it is more indicative of a primary depressive disorder if the patient and his family cannot, try as they may, come up with a plausible precipitant. They have to conclude that as far as they can see the depression "came out of the blue" and that "he has no reason to be this way." It is equally significant when they say that nothing they do seems to "snap him out of it.,"

In a sense, this primary depressive disorder displays neither "causing" nor "treating" precipitants such as stresses, disasters and bad news or, on the other hand, gifts, attention or even threats. The depression displays an endogenous characteristic and is seemingly intent on running an autonomous course which is independent of major external influences.

Whether the proposed precipitants are the cause or the result of the depressive disorder, the fact remains that they are of major clinical significance in the overall clinical picture. Despite their role, the stresses must be dealt with in an appropriate manner. Factors such as loss of employment, economic crises, marital strife and alcoholism may be the most pressing issues at the time of presentation regardless of whether they have a primary or secondary character. Even if the medical student's examination failure was the result of a longstanding and unrecognised depressive disorder, it is wrong to conclude that treatment simply involves the prescribing of an antidepressant.

All cases must be approached from a combined biological, psychological and sociological viewpoint in order for the treatment to have its maximum effect. Medications, such as antidepressants, are very effective when given an adequate therapeutic trial but they are not "happy pills" or "magic solvers of life's problems." Unfortunately, perhaps because of the erroneous equating of the depressive symptom to the depressive syndrome, these medications are increasingly misused as "passive solutions to unhappiness."

5. Alteration in Cognition

Typically, the depressed patient complains of a slowness of thinking with a poverty of productive ideation. Frequently, this is expressed by the patient as an inability to remember events and recall information. This memory impairment can present akin to dementia. However, this is not the primary dementia seen in organic brain syndromes but rather an impaired recall due to difficulties in concentration and holding a mental set.

The differentiation of memory impairment due to major depressive disorder and that due to organic brain syndrome is of particular concern in geriatric patients. It is necessary to rule out a major affective disorder in elderly patients who present with memory impairment and other features suggestive of dementia. One condition is very likely to show a response to treatment whereas the other may be irreversible.

The patient with a major depressive episode is likely to become overconcerned and preoccupied with depressive material. This preoccupation may develop into ruminations which can dominate the patient's mental state. A paralysis of the person's cognitive function can result. The ruminations may take the form of a search for a cause or reason for the dysphoria ending in "the dog chasing its tail."

This ruminative ongoing and non-productive internal debate may produce desperate and pathetic fabrications such as "this is all due to my cheating on my income tax forty-two years ago." This notion may become fixed as a conviction in the person's mental state. Many patients, feeling they are being deservedly punished for past transgressions, show a quality of resignation towards their predicament. There is associated guilt, feelings of worthlessness and growing interminable anguish.

The ruminations may develop into obsessions. The patients experience a persistant intrusion of unwanted and anxiety provoking thoughts relating to their condition, for example, reasons for their depression and hopelessness. Attempts at momentary relief from this intrapsychic turmoil can result in compulsive behavior which further impairs their condition. The appearance of obsessive-compulsive symptoms at thirty and forty years of age should result in the consideration of an underlying major depressive disorder as the possible etiology. It should be recalled that these obsessive-compulsive symptoms can be the dominant symptom of the clinical presentation of a major affective disorder.

Patients suffering from a major depressive disorder have problems maintaining a cognitive set. Clearly, the presence of preoccupations, ruminations and obsessions will prove to be detrimental. The person's concentration span will be disrupted and on clinical examination or psychometric testing he will show memory impairment.

Cognitive function can be impaired and give rise to formal thought disorders. These can include the types discussed earlier in connection with the schizophrenias, for example, overinclusivity, tangentiality and derailment as well as circumstantiality and interpenetration of themes. It is probable that the content of these thought disorders will display a depressive quality. Symptoms such as thought blocking, withdrawal, insertion and diffusion also may arise in the cognitive dysfunction of a major depressive disorder.

This situation can lead to symptoms of paranoid ideation. Instead of acknowledging a growing ineffectiveness at work due to reduced mental quickness, memory impairment and anergia, the depressed patient may conclude that his workmates are hostile and presecutory. Rather than recognising that his family is at a loss in dealing with his depressive syndrome, the patient may decide that they are abandoning or shunning him.

This mixture of pathological and non-pathological processes within the mental state resulting in intrapsychic turmoil may first manifest as a change in the patient's basic personality. The habitual traits which characterise the individual's personality may become ones of suspiciousness, hypervigilance and a readiness to ascribe ill intent to others. This situation is ripe for misinterpretations, ideas of reference and a plethora of secondary verifications which compound the disorder.

A change in personality and lifestyle to one of the paranoid type may be the dominant clinical feature of an affective disorder's presentation. As with all paranoid states, whether of functional or toxic etiology, the major affective disorders can give rise to a primary delusion. The content of a primary delusion due to a major affective disorder is not limited to being persecutory. For example, as a response to the marked loss of self-esteem, the depressed patient may develop a grandiose delusional content. The delusional content may be religious, litigious, erotic or somatic but one with a persecutory flavour is more likely.

In some cases of the major depressive syndrome of *involutional melancholia,* a primary delusion arises which is characteristically somatic in nature. The patients are convinced, for example, that their bowels have "turned to concrete," their brains have "turned to dust" or that their bodies are being "eaten away by cancer." There may be accompanying congruent hallucinations such as feeling the cancer invading the brain or smelling the bodies decay. Often, these notions are accepted with a resignation, for example, the patients can conclude that the cancerous decay is justly deserved and a fitting punishment for past transgressions. The somatic delusions have a *nihilistic* quality with feelings of negation, futility and a lack of meaning to the worth and meaning of life. In short, life is "a walking shadow full of sound and fury signifying nothing."

6. Alteration in Energy

Frequently, patients with a major depressive disorder complain of weakness, fatigue and loss of enthusiasm. It is an effort to even think about, let alone carry out, simple tasks. These *neurasthenic* symptoms of physical and mental exhaustion can progress to a retarded catatonic state and depressive stupor.

There is often a deterioration in work performance, a loss of interest in family and pasttimes and a decreased socialisation. The family may press activities on the patient in the hope of 'snapping him out of it" but this is likely to fail and simply aggravate the difficulties and increase the patient's despair. Sending the patient on an ocean cruise is not the correct intervention in a major depressive disorder.

In this progressively anergic condition, the feelings of hopelessness, worthlessness and guilt will further develop. In a state of depressive stupor, a suicidal patient may be anergic to the point of being unable to carry through a suicidal act but it should be noted that as this depressive state lifts the risk of suicide increases.

7. Hypochondriasis

Psychodynamically, a central feature of depression is a loss of self-esteem. A preoccupation with physical ailments may be thought of as a partial defense against feelings of inadequacy, ineffectiveness and lowered self-esteem.

Hypochondriasis is usually defined as an overconcern and preoccupation with physical ailments in the absense of demonstrable organic pathology. Referring to a person as being hypochondrical, usually carries with it a perjorative connotation. This categorization is often used as a means of "turfing" a tiresome patient. It should be borne in mind that stating there is no organic pathology requires that one has first carefully investigated all the possibilities.

It is not that there is no pathology associated with hypochondriasis but rather that the organic damage if it is present is slight and does not warrant the patient's distress and disability. For example, the patient may have mild diabetes or episodic cystitis which then becomes an exaggerated focus of attention in the depressed state. Overconcern and preoccupation may result in the patient worrying that his diabetes mellitus is the beginning of a neuroendocrine disaster or the cystitis is an early symptom of malignant bladder cancer.

The concerns about physical problems provide a tangible "cause" for the patient's other difficulties and this explanation is more acceptable to the patient and to others than is "depression." The feelings of inadequacy, hopelessness, and despair are palatable since, after all, the person and others sees him as "really sick." The hypochondriasis lessens the need to be aware of other issues which will lessen self-esteem.

The depressed patient, not necessarily displaying sadness or the blues, may "doctor shop" in an attempt to justify and obtain treatment for his impairment and thereby continue this "diversionary" tactic. If he does not receive satisfaction, he may question the doctor's competency which can increase the likelihood of a "turf." Many of these patients become sophisticated in medical matters, asking, for example, 'What percentage of epileptic activity fails to be recorded on a single EEG tracing, doctor?" or "Maybe my duodenal ulcer was poorly visualised by the last GI series that I had, doctor?"

Classically, the organ system focused on by the hypochondriasis symptoms of major depressive disorders is the gastrointestinal tract. Certainly the interaction between the mental state and disorders such as peptic ulcers and inflammatory bowel disease is apparent to all clinicians. Since these hypochondriasis features can be the dominant presenting symptom of a major depressive disorder, one has to wonder what percentage of patients diagnosed as having an irritable bowel syndrome had, in fact, a major depressive disorder which went unrecognised.

Recent studies report the success of some antidepressants in the treatment of peptic ulcers and bowel diseases such as ulcerative colitis. They focus on the histamine receptor blocking properties of these drugs. It is interesting that these receptors are found in the brain as well as the bowel and that histamine has the properties of a neurotransmitter. Therefore, is the antidepressant treating the primary bowel symptom or is it treating the primary depression which has an association gastrointestional problem? After all, a major component of ulcer therapy is to tell the patient not to get so emotionally distraught in addition to taking antacids.

A very important manifestation of hypochondriasis is pain. The word is derived from the Greek "poine" meaning penalty. It should not matter whether or not the clinician can find a "real" source for the patient's pain, what is at issue is the patient's evaluation of pain and his need to focus on the phenomena. After all, in the final analysis, pain is a mental pheonomenon which depends on the person's mental state at that time. A reduction in pain following an injection of normal saline proves little in terms of whether or not the patient has "real" pain. One can relieve, somewhat, the pain of an acute myocardial simply by giving the patient attention and reassurance. In the vast majority of instances these injections are more revealing about the doctor than the patient.

8. Depersonnalization, Derealization

Derealization can present as nihilism and negation, with the world being perceived as "gray and dark without warmth or colour." In a milder form, derealization may be expressed as "Things are not the same, I do not see the world like I used to."

Perception can be disturbed in a major depressive disorder giving rise to misperceptions, illusions and hallucinations. A sleep disturbance with long periods of light sleep increases the likelihood of hypnogogic and hyponopompic hallucinations. In grief reactions, many people "see" their dead relative during the course of a disturbed sleep or hear him in the bedroom on a few isolated occasions.

Depersonnalization may involve feelings of being ouside of one's body or not being in control of one's thinking or actions. These may develop into passivity symptoms of the type discussed in connection with the schizophrenias. Dysmorphobic delusions, which refer to somatic changes, such as the body decaying or rotting, were mentioned earlier and have features of depersonnalization. Usually, these symptoms have a content which is congruent with the other characteristics of the dysphoria and so compound and enlarge the clinical problem.

9. Sexual Interests

Generally, sexual activity is decreased in depressive disorders. This will likely add to feelings of worthlessness and increase loss of self-esteem. The decrease is not restricted to performance and frequency but includes, perhaps more significantly, interest, motivation and desire.

Sexual dysfunction can be the presenting symptom of a depressive syndrome. This is well borne in mind by family practitioners. It may be a source of rumination with guilt being ascribed to long past and minimal indiscretions which may in turn be pathologically reasoned as the "cause" of the problem. The vast majority of sexual dysfunction is of functional or psychological etiology.

10. Dysphoria

Symptoms of dysphoria are frequently, though by no means always, prominent in the clinical presentation of major depressive disorder. However, it cannot be overemphasized that the presence of symptoms such as depression, sadness and unhappiness does not necessarily mean the presence of a major depressive disorder. To stress this crucial point, dysphoria has been placed at the end of this list of symptoms rather than at the beginning.

The dysphoria of a depressive syndrome has a variety of manifestations. A common symptom, which may well dominate the affective component, is anxiety. This free-floating tension, apprehension and fear is likely to be present to some degree in all depressive disorders. Other dysphoria features include sadness, unhappiness, despondency, perplexity and with the patient devoid of any emotional tone and unable to comprehend an affect, let alone feel or express one.

It is possible that even with the presence of the whole range of symptoms currently outlined in this list, a major depressive syndrome may be dominated by, for example, obsessive-compulsive symptoms, a primary delusion or cognitive impairment with little apparent sadness in the clinical presentation.

Clearly, the eliciting of the above symptoms must be viewed as a group and in context with the absence of symptoms which are characteristic of other disorder in the differential diagnosis. Additional information, such as details of previous psychiatric illness, is important. The nature of the symptoms of these previous disorders, their course, response to various treatments and the outcome aid in the clarification of the clinical diagnosis.

Details regarding the patient's family history of psychiatric disorders is helpful. As will be discussed in a later chapter, the primary affective disorders have notable genetic and familial characteristics.

A comprehensive developmental history including educational, social, occupational and marital details is informative. This helps to outline the natural course of the premorbid state and points to the person's coping mechanisms, strengths and weaknesses. It also indicates the psycho-social circumstances of the given patient and helps in formulating a comprehensive treatment plan.

Finally, the past and present medical history is crucial. There are many disorders which can begin their clinical presentation in the form suggestive of a depressive disorder. Many of these disorders, even when fully developed, can have a clinical presentation which is dominated by symptoms characteristic of a major depressive illness. The important question of primary versus secondary depressive disorders must be considered at all times. The medications which have been prescribed or taken for many other medical conditions can mimic the symptoms of major depressive disorders.

DESCRIPTIVE ASPECTS OF MANIA

The clinical features of mania can be grouped as the "3 a's." The similarity to the Bleulerian "4 a's" is intentional in order to stress the lack of pathognomonic symptoms of the principal functional psychoses.

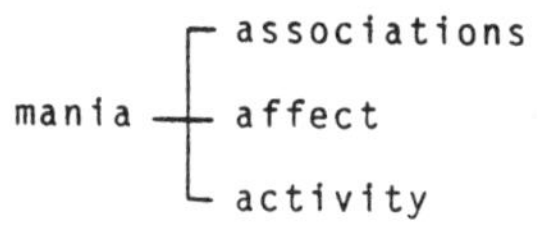

Figure 33

The cardinal symptoms arising from a disturbance of cognition are grouped under associations. The motor and behavioural abnormalities seen in mania are grouped under activity, and the affect group is self-explanatory.

The following symptom subheadings are not listed in order of frequency or importance. The similarity to the previous listing for depression indicates the commonality of etiology, namely, a central disturbance of mood. In a particular case, some of the following symptoms may not be present and the dominating symptoms can very with time.

1. Alteration in Sleep

Invariably in mania there is a marked reduction in the patient's total sleep time. Characteristically the manic is able to function, though pathologically in many respects, on a few hours of sleep per night for an extended period of time.

Classically, the patient shows terminal insomnia with an abrupt awakening in the early morning hours. Understandably, a frequent chief complaint of the patient's family refers to the patient's insomnia. Significantly, hypnotics usually do not adequately alleviate this symptom. In fact, it is unlikely that the manic will take such medication since he does not require more sleep.

Initial insomnia is also seen in mania. The patient's various forms of hyperactivity can extend well into the night much to dismay of his family and associates. As is the case in major depression, the duration of the sleep is not the issue as much as the quality of sleep required by the patient.

The EEG recorded during sleep in manic patients shows a disruption from the normal pattern. There is a disturbance of the normal sleep stages, with both REM and non-REM stages being reduced. However, the manics appear to "protect" themselves to a degree by "cramming" the key stages into the overall reduced sleep time. For example, although there is some reduction in the time spent in non-REM Stage 4, this is quite small and its percentage of the total sleep time is increased over the normal percentage. This compensation is not totally successful and over a period of weeks most manics will begin to show fatigue-related problems.

2. Alteration in Appetite

Classically, the appetite is increased. However, because of the patient's distractability and hyperactivity the actual food intake is not increased. In fact, in most cases, the intake is decreased and there is a weight loss. It is unlikely that this decrease in weight can be accounted for by the patient's overactivity "burning off the calories." The manic may persistently demand food, but by the time it arrives, he may have moved on to a more absorbing project, forgetting the meal.

Frequently, there is an increased appetite for alcohol and this is very often satisfied. The result is a further increase in some of the patient's symptomatology. As in the case of the depression, the manic's actions and behaviour lead to a compounding of the underlying problems and symptomatology.

3. Diurnal Variation

Both the patient and staff describe a variation in the manic's mood throughout the day. Classically, the mood is at its most labile and "euphoric" in the early part of the day. Often, it is the evening shift which first notices the mood coming back to baseline with the day shift being the last to report this improvement.

As with the depressive diurnal variation, the manic's mood change is more than a simple reflection of the stressors encountered during the day. Wards tend to be at their most hectic in the mornings and the manic's distractability, lability and impulsivity would be expected to escalate in this period. If the manic is placed in a seclusion room, this diurnal pattern decreases but is still present and displays autonomous and endogeneously derived fluctuations.

Mania has a "cascade" process of responding to events, thereby eliciting responses which in turn become events to react to. In such an escalating situation, the role of stressors and precipitants in etiological sense of primary versus secondary is difficult to ascertain but that it exists is patently obvious.

4. Precipitants

In contrast to many patients with major depressive disorders, the manic does not become seclusive and withdrawn. At the time of hospitalisation, it is likely that the history will contain and feature many factors which could be precipitants in the disorder.

When these factors are viewed in the time frame of the developing mania, it is frequently seen that they are responses because of the mania rather than its "cause." Precipitants as a necessary and sufficient primary etiology of mania are less conclusive than in the depressive phase of a major affective disorder.

Nevertheless, these "secondary" precipitants will undoubtably escalate the clinical presentation and will be a major factor in the final outcome of the mania episode. For example, a person in the middle of a manic episode may lose a great deal of money during a trip to Las Vegas, and they did not become manic because they went there, but the clinical facts are unlikely to carry much weight with the collection agency.

5. Alterations in Cognition

There is a marked problem in maintaining a cognitive set. This is due to loosening of associations and a lessening of internal constraints along the same lines discussed earlier in connection with the schizophrenias. Also, the manic exhibits marked distractability and overinclusivity for events that occur in his environment which adds to the cognitive difficulties. As a result, the formal thought disorder in mania is frequently more florrid and dramatic than that seen in schizophrenias.

The external distractability means that an examiner can "plant cues" as the manic is talking and 'lead" the patient's interpretation of themes, tangentiality and derailment. Therefore, the resulting pressure of speech and flight of ideas can have some degree of meaning to the observer because of these deliberate reference points.

The manic can become overconcerned and preoccupied to the point of ruminating and when this is coupled with the formal thought disorder the result can be agitated stereotypies. Essentially, the manic is "spinning his wheels" to the point of non-function. Clearly, there is a need to work through an adequate toxic-organic differential diagnosis.

The attention span is particularly short because of the formal thought disorder and the labile mood. This is invariably frustrating for the patient and results in him becoming irritable, sarcastic and "nasty." A serene state of grace is rare.

In coping with this intrapsychic dysequilibrium, the the manic is very likely to employ projection. Grandiosity, like persecution, has projection as its basic mechanism. Notions of persecution often soon follow those of grandiosity since they explain why the special gifts and abilities have not been recognised or rewarded. Misinterpretations, paranoid ideation and ideas of reference of a persecutory, litigious, somatic, erotic and religious nature can occur in connection with the original grandiose material.

Primary delusions arise in mania from a pathological cognitive set which is congruent and internally consistent with the other sets and components comprising the mental state. Delusions of grandiose content can arise in any psychotic disorder whether of functional or toxic-organic etiology. Pure grandiose delusions of a sustained type are rare in mania since it is very likely that other content, such as persecutory and litigious, will be added to the grandiosity.

6. Alteration in Energy

Invariably, the overall energy level is elevated but when coupled with the association and affect abnormalities it is not effective in a productive manner. There is a lack of application due to failure in following through tasks because of the short attention span and impulsivity. However, in the early phase of mania, the productivity in certain spheres may be increased and effective before the disruptive aspects of mania interfere. For example, in the early stages, so-called *hypomania,* the individual may be a successful travelling salesman.

The coupling of this high energy to the association, affect and activity symptoms will become a liability for the manic and others. Impulsive, disinhibited and ill-considered behaviour such as the classic spending sprees, business ventures and alcoholism frequently give rise to tragic difficulties. There is a limit in the ability to psychologically and physiologically "burn the candle at both ends."

In some cases, the energy level shows periods of relative anergia. This is a reflection of the fluctuation and lability of mania. Although the retarded period is short lived, there is a risk of suicide during this time and anergia should not be taken as a sign of the manic being "cured."

7. Alteration in Perception

Misperceptions, illusions and hallucinations can occur in mania as the core perturbation extends into the perception component of the mental state. These can take a Schneiderian first rank form and when coupled with some specific cognitive symptoms the differentiation of mania from schizophrenia or schizophreniform disorders is difficult.

Obviously, the occurrence of these perception symptoms places a drug toxic state high in the differential diagnosis of acute mania. Clinically, the level of consciousness can present with impairment but the problem is to decide whether this is primary or secondary alteration. Since mania often leads to substance abuse, the likelihood of a combination of primary and secondary changes in the level of consciousness is high.

8. Sexual Interests

The sexual appetite, like its nutritional counterpart, is increased. In severe mania, there is a chance that the sexual appetite will not be satisfied because of the overall disruption of association, affect and activity. However, in the earlier phase of mania or in less severe cases, the disinhibition and impulsivity may result in numerous sexual problems. The wives of male manics can be harassed and brutalised severely by their husbands.

9. Substance Abuse

In mania, this warrants special mention. The abuse of alcohol in depression may or may not be present to a significant degree but in mania it is very likely a factor of major concern. In the milder phase of mania, the "hail fellow well met" characteristics and "life in the fast lane" lend so well to substance abuse.

In primary affective disorders, particularly the bipolar type, a positive family history of alcoholism is very often the case. The bipolar disorders and alcoholism are intertwined such that functional manic symptoms are often reported as being "due to his drinking" and a family history of mania or depression is misunderstood by relatives.

10. Dysphoria

This is a cardinal feature of mania but it must not be assumed that all manics are euphoric and all euphorics are manic. Classically, the dysphoria of mania is one of exuberance, elation and euphoria. However, irritability, anxiety, anger, frustration and despondency can all be prominent features of this condition.

A crucial feature of manic dysphoria is its lability, fluctuation and impulsivity. It is possible to see the "emotional incontinence" which is classically associated with the organic frontal lobe syndrome. The explosive and catastrophic emotional outbursts which are apparently unrelated to adequate triggering seen in this brain syndrome are well represented in functional mania.

The manic's frustrations can lead to profound anger, sarcasm and "nastiness." The manic affect is said to be "infectious" which at times makes the patient "amusing and funny." If this is the case, it is either likely to be shortlived or in a patient with a mild version of this disorder. Primary or "full blown" mania is not cute.

Clearly, the elliciting of the above symptoms must be assessed in context with the absence of symptoms which are characteristic of other disorders in the differential diagnosis. Additional information, such as details of previous psychiatric illness, is important. The nature of the symptoms of these previous disorders, their course, response to various treatments and the outcome aid in the clarification of the clinical diagnosis.

Details regarding the patient's family history of psychiatric disorders are helpful. As will be discussed in a later chapter, the primary affective disorders have notable genetic and familial characteristics.

A comprehensive developmental history including educational, social, occupational and marital details is informative. This helps to outline the natural course of the premorbid state and points to the person's coping mechanisms, strengths and weaknesses. It also indicates the psycho-social circumstances of the given patient and helps in formulating a comprehensive treatment plan.

Finally, the past and present medical history is crucial. There are many disorders which can begin their clinical presentation in the form suggestive of a manic disorder. Many of these disorders, even when fully developed, can have a clinical presentation which is dominated by symptoms characteristic of a major affective disorder. The important question of primary versus secondary affective disorders must be considered at all times. The medications which have been prescribed or taken for many other medical conditions can mimic the symptoms of mania.

CHAPTER 12

THE SUBTYPES OF MAJOR AFFECTIVE DISORDERS

The symptomatology and some diagnostic classifications of the major affective disorders have been outlined in the previous chapter. Using this information the formal major clinical subtypes will now be outlined along with three special clinical syndromes, namely, involutional melancholia, postpartum disorders and grief reactions.

BIPOLAR DISORDERS

As seen in Figure 31, the bipolar disorders are a sub-type of primary affective disorders. By definition, these patients do not have a current or past history of disorders requiring the diagnosis of a secondary affective disorder.

The natural course of a bipolar disorder has episodes of either a depressive or a manic type. These episodes, namely, *bipolar disorder, manic phase* and *bipolar disorder, depressed phase,* are shown schematically in Figure 32 b.

The formal diagnosis of a bipolar manic phase needs to either have been sustained for at least one week or sufficiently debilitating and severe that hospitalisation is necessary within that time. The bipolar depressive phase needs to have been sustained for at least two weeks.

One of the reasons to impose time periods on the episodes stems from the fact that the secondary affective disorders, for example, an adult adjustment disorder due to a severe marital dispute, can acutely present with an array of symptoms characteristic of primary affective disorders. Appropriate psycho-social intervention may alleviate these symptoms, such as initial and terminal insomnia, loss of appetite, profound dysphoria and suicidal thoughts, within a matter of days.

Many toxic-organic disorders, for example, alcoholism and abuse of anxiolytics, can result in secondary affective disorders which significantly differ at the time of presentation from the primary affective disorders only in terms of the mode of onset and duration. Nevertheless, the one and two week stipulations should not be taken too literally or applied too rigourously. For instance, a five day duration of depression does not rule out a primary depressive disorder nor is treatment "withheld" to see if the episode will run the defined period.

What is seen as a primary affective disorder at the time of admission may turn out to be a secondary affective disorder when more history becomes available. Similarly, what is taken as an adult adjustment disorder at hospitalisation may turn out to be superimposed and the result of an underlying bipolar or unipolar disorder. Frequently, with additional laboratory data and clinical history, there is a need to revise the admission diagnosis.

In addition to bipolar disorder, manic phase and bipolar disorder, depressed phase, there is a third subgroup, namely, *bipolar disorder, mixed phase.* As the name implies, this phase has both manic and depressive symptoms coexisting in the current clinical presentation.

CYCLOTHYMIC DISORDER

The onset of bipolar disorders can follow a variety of profiles over time. Some patients rapidly develop a "full blown" clinical profile whilst others slowly manifest the profile of a bipolar disorder. There are others who never manifest the "full blown" bipolar spectrum or severity of symptoms but instead have a "muted" expression of the disorder.

The *cyclothymic disorder* can be viewed as a partial or "hypo" expression of the bipolar disorder. At some later date in the clinical course, a complete bipolar episode may arise but for many patients the cyclothymic disorder remains as the clinical presentation.

These patients have mild manic and depressive episodes extending over the years. Isolated symptoms characteristic of the bipolar phase can occur but the patients do not manifest bipolar symptoms such as delusions, hallucinations or profound thought disorders.

In some cases, the cyclothymic patient "swings" rapidly from mild depression to mild mania and vice-versa. This oscillation may have a short periodicity measured in days rather than the weeks and months seen in bipolar disorders. The result of the *rapid cycling* is that the patients have great difficulty regulating their lives. The personality which develops under these precarious circumstances is often, and understandably, problematic in many respects.

Precipitants for the rapid cyclic mood invariably cannot be found. This autonomous quality of the dysphoria and associated symptoms is similar to that seen in bipolar disorders. The result is that the person operates in an unpredictable state so much so that many of these patients consider that a mildly depressed but stable mood would be preferable to the oscillating type.

It should be stressed that in many respects the cyclothymic disorder is as debilitating as the "full blown" bipolar disorder. The milder degree of symptomatology means that patients with the cyclothymic disorder phases may go unnoticed and untreated for a long time. In general, severe and dramatic disorders lead to intervention but a "smoldering" illness can be overlooked with a resulting accruement of crippling symptoms.

In order to emphasize this point, it is helpful to refer to an older diagnostic entity called the *emotionally unstable character disorder.* This is not related to the bipolar disorder but has a number of similarities with the bipolar related cyclothymic disorder.

In the emotionally unstable character disorder, precipitating factors for changes in the person's mood are readily apparent. The pathological characteristic is that minimal stresses give rise to extreme fluctuations in the person's mood. The name of the syndrome says it all: they are emotionally unstable. They "fall apart and take to their beds" with minimal provocation or become "crazily delighted" with slight praise. In short, they have a tendency to "go off the deep end." These people find it difficult to "keep a roommate."

As in the case of the bipolar related cyclothymic disorder, these people lead a precarious existence. There is much social disruption for them and others due to the oversensitivity and overactivity. The likelihood of having treatment is probably less than in the case of the cyclothymic disorders but the disruption in personality development and interpersonal relationship is extreme.

UNIPOLAR DISORDER

By definition, this is a primary affective disorder. The difference between bipolar and unipolar disorders is that the latter does not have evidence of a current or past manic episode. All episodes in a unipolar disorder will be depressive in nature. As in the case of the bipolar disorder, depressed phase, the formal diagnosis of a unipolar episode requires a duration of at least two weeks.

DYSTHYMIC DISORDER

The *dysthymic disorder* corresponds to the unipolar disorder as the cyclothymic relates to the bipolar disorder.

A fairly steady mild depressive syndrome occurs over a period of years. Short periods of normal mood can be seen during this extended period, but in general the patient operates from a depressed position.

The reactivity of the patient to his overall circumstances and environment, along with the subsequent reaction of other people to him, leads to a complicated clinical presentation. It is in this disorder, probably more so than in any other affective illness, that presents difficulties in sorting out the biological, psychological and sociological factors which comprise the clinical presentation.

It is likely that psycho-social factors have intertwined into the clinical picture over a prolonged period of dysthymia. Although the dysthymic disorder is a "strain" of the unipolar disorder, it is highly unlikely that antidepressants will be the major therapeutic intervention.

INVOLUTIONAL MELANCHOLIA

Primary depressive disorders often go unrecognised or misdiagnosed in the elderly patient. Symptoms of psychomotor retardation and intellectual impairment are easily taken as diagnostic of a chronic organic brain syndrome. If there are accompanying abnormalities on a CT scan or an EEG, then the likelihood of a diagnosis of chronic organic brain syndrome is greatly increased. However, it should be noted that these abnormalities may simply be related to normal aging and have little or no clinical significance in regard to the psychomotor and intellectual difficulties.

The syndrome of *involutional melancholia* can be adequately classified as a unipolar depression in the elderly. However, it has the clinical importance to warrant a separate discussion. The tragic overlooking of depressive disorders in geriatrics warrants emphasis of syndromes such as involutional melancholia to the point of belabourment.

Involutional melancholia has its presentation in late middle age, the involuntional period. This disorder is more common in women than in men by some three to one. For these patients, it usually represents their first psychiatric episode which requires clinical intervention. The onset is characteristically insidious without noticeable necessary and sufficient precipitants.

The early phase is characterised by an agitated dysphoria. There is a general loss of interests, and often there will be a deterioration in the patients habits and behaviour. Usually, insomnia is the first indication of the disorder. During the daytime, the patient becomes anxious and restless with pacing, wringing of hands and non-specific pleas for help and reassurance.

Feelings of helplessness and anxiety increase leading to pervasive notions of hopelessness, worthlessness and guilt. Self-directed accusations, condemnations and incriminations result in pathetic fabrication of events deemed responsible for the turmoil. The patient is often resigned to this intrapsychic turmoil and although this is "painful," it is felt to be a punishment well-deserved.

The decompensation can be accompanied by features of derealisation and depersonalization. The patient's "world" is perceived with a sense of negation and devoid of meaning or value. Misinterpretations, illusions and hallucinations can occur which are congruent with the core affect disturbance and the overall problems are compounded. Trivial problems, difficulties and concerns become distorted by the onset of paranoid ideation.

Medical problems, often of a trivial nature, can form a focus for hypochondrical symptoms or these concerns can develop in the absence of organ pathology. Dysmorphobic delusions, such as pathological convictions that the body is decaying, infected, cancerous or is already "dead," can arise. This subgroup of involutional melancholia which features somatic delusions and nihilism is Cotard's syndrome.

Involutional melancholia comes at an age which is for many people a time of personal reflection and evaluation. One "asks" whether the previous decades have involved stagnation or generation and whether the future is to be of integrity or despair.

The individual's socio-cultural values can prove to be problematic at this time. For example, the person may conclude a devastating loss of "virility" which is not restricted to the sexual sense. The young can be viewed as a threat to their security and position. Both men and women can experience a numbing sense of loss in prestige, self-esteem and self-worth. There is a painful questioning of their past and future roles within the changing family structure and society. The threat of "menopause" and the "empty nest" syndrome are not exclusive to females unless one mistakenly views the problem in terms of simple hormones and housekeeping.

The neuroendocrinological aspects of the major psychiatric disorders at this time in life is a complex issue. It is naive to consider that involutional melancholia is simply related to changes in estrogen, progesterone and their neuronal precursors. For example, estrogen replacement for "hot flashes" at the "change of life" may often produce a placebo response rather than a neuroendocrine benefit and the physiological problems are only the "tip of the iceberg."

Classically, the premorbid personality of those who develop involutional melancholia is of the obsessive-compulsive type. In most instances, this type of personality has served the person well over the years. It is often surprising to relatives that these previously active, powerful and controlling individuals succumb to such doubts and fears in late middle age. However, the "double den mother" may take the departure of her children for college as "the end" of her useful and meaningful life and may be unable to find anything to fill the void. Similarly, a man may take retirement to be the end of his usefulness and productivity. In both instances, there has been a loss of many of the factors which provided the person with self-esteem and a role in the hierarchy.

Patients with involutional melancholia will likely have a poor score on psychometric testing. If this finding occurs along with agitation, psychotic symptoms such as a delusion, and an affect which is labile and anxious, then the misdiagnosis of organic brain syndrome with psychotic features is likely.

Late onset schizophrenia, that is to say, paraphrenia, is a diagnosis which is likely to be considered. After all, depersonalization, derealization, illusions, hallucinations, paranoid ideation and primary delusions are possible in the clinical presentation of paraphrenia. The fact that the involutional melancholic's agitation and anxiety may partially respond to neuroleptics may be incorrectly taken as "proof" of an underlying schizophrenic process by the illinformed clinician.

It is necessary to work through a comprehensive toxic-organic differential diagnosis in these patients. One of these disorders may well be the etiology of the mental disorder, but if not, it can still contribute, if present, to the psychiatric problems. The elderly, particularly with a mental disorder as part of the presentation, tend to receive poor medical attention. For many, this toxic-organic work-up as part of their psychiatric evaluation may well be their first medical assessment in years.

Involutional melancholia has a notable mortality. In one study, this was given as 40 percent. This is not simply due to the accompanying disorders to which the elderly are more prone. Severe involutional melancholia can result in agitated catatonia with verbal and motor stereotypies which leads to physical and mental exhaustion. Secondary medical complications resulting from the mental symptoms will increase the morbidity and mortality risk in these patients.

Biological treatment involving neuroleptics may be required in order to quickly reduce the patient's agitation and allow basic nursing to be given. However, treating the underlying affective etiology requires the use of antidepressants or convulsive therapy (ECT). The antidepressants have a number of relative contraindications, such as cardiovascular problems, which are likely to be present in the elderly. A major draw back is that these drugs can take weeks to be maximumly effective and there is a need for rapid intervention in the treatment of involutional melancholia. Under such circumstances, the treatment of choice is convulsive therapy (ECT). These points concerning antidepressants and ECT will be discussed in detail later in the text.

Psycho-social intervention is mandatory in conjunction with the somatic therapies. There must be a reassessment and clarification of values, expectations and circumstances of both the patient and his family. The recovery from involutional melancholia can be one of the most dramatic and satisfying to be witnessed in psychiatry. Perhaps its only draw back is to realise how many patients with this reversible disorder are not correctly diagnosed and treated.

POSTPARTUM DISORDERS

Psychiatric problems related to giving birth to a child have been recorded in one form or another for centuries. Although the number of the toxic-organic related difficulties has been reduced by modern obstetrical techniques, the incidence of associated psychiatric problems remains high. A major factor in determining the incidence of these problems is the vigilance and awareness of the attending physician.

The incidence of postpartum "baby blues" has been recorded, by various studies, from five to eighty percent of deliveries. This wide range indicates the diversity of presentation as well as pointing to a range of clinical awareness.

In general, the "baby blues" occurs within two to three days of delivery but there is a notable delay of some twenty-four hours following delivery. Typically, the onset features fatigue and oversensitivity in the mother with anxiety regarding her future role as a parent. The concerns about mothering cover a whole spectrum of psycho-social and biological issues. It should be borne in mind that many parents are poorly prepared for their role.

The precipitous drop in the level of a number of hormones and their precursors at the time of delivery has led to many neuroendrocrinological investigations of a possible etiological role. However, as in the case of involutional melancholia and premenstrual tension, the findings have, for the most part, been inconclusive.

In general, the "baby blues" are considered to be a common and relatively benign occurrence in the peuperium. The problem usually spontaneously resolves within several days or a couple of weeks. Treatment consists of direct psycho-social support and there is usually no need for medications.

If the "baby blues" continue for a number of weeks, the possibility of a *postpartum depression* should be considered. Once again, the incidence of this disorder depends on the diagnostic awareness of the attending physician. The incidence of postpartum depression is a couple of percent of all deliveries by a consensus of studies.

In addition to the features of the "baby blues," some of the characteristic symptoms of a major depressive disorder are present in postpartum depression. There is a wide range of symptoms, and common findings include somatic complaints, irritability and lability of mood, suspiciousness and paranoid ideation.

The postpartum depression can develop symptoms seen with a primary depressive disorder which requires an adequate trial of antidepressant medications in addition to psycho-social intervention. Typically, the onset of the postpartum depression is some two to three weeks after delivery. This significant delay is one of the reasons for this syndrome frequently going unrecognised. Obviously, the likelihood of overlooking this diagnosis is increased if the clinician considers major depressive illness to be synonymous with sadness, weeping and despondency.

If a major depressive episode begins more than three months after delivery, then it is taken to be unrelated to the birth of the child.

Understandably, attempts have been made to identify factors which place mothers at a higher risk of having a postpartum depression. Various personality profiles and psycho-social stressors have been noted in patients who developed postpartum depressions. However, these profiles and stress inventories were formulated retrospectively and do not have the desired predictive value of identifying high-risk mothers prior to giving birth. If a pregnant woman has a previous psychiatric history, in particular a primary affective disorder, she ought to be closely followed during the pregnancy and postpartum. It must be noted that women are at their greatest risk of presenting with a primary affective disorder during the childbearing years. A previous history of major depressive illness is the most valid indicator of the at-risk mother.

It was stressed earlier in the text that a very useful piece of information aiding in the diagnosis of primary affective disorder is the patients past psychiatric history. An important line of questioning in this regard concerns the postpartum history. Usually, hospital records are of little help but questions such as "Were you able to bounce back and look after the baby?" can lead to information suggesting a more severe version of the "baby blues."

Postpartum disorders can arise in the form of brief reactive psychoses of schizophreniform-like disorders. These are often referred to as *postpartum psychoses.* The full range of symptoms for the brief reactive psychoses and schizophreniform disorders, discussed earlier in the text, can be seen following the birth of a child. However, the appearance of isolated psychotic symptoms in the post-partum period does not exclude postpartum depression as the problem. Also, the appearance of psychotic symptoms makes it important to rule out *postpartum delerium disorders* of toxic-organic etiology.

GRIEF REACTIONS

Periods of bereavement and grief will occur in everyone's life. Ironically, in many instances, it is the lack of grief and bereavement that is more indicative of problems.

The perceived loss of an important object relation, for example, a sibling, spouse or friend, results in intrapsychic turmoil. It was pointed out earlier in the text that an object relation does not refer to the visual-spatial properties of an object but rather to its representation within the mental set by an ascribed affect. Furthermore, the object relation can be "things" such as ambition, values and principles as well as people.

The restoration of intrapsychic equilibrium following an object loss requires a *working through* of aspects associated with the lost object with a reintegration of associated mental processes. A grief reaction, with distortion of mental processes due to the intrapsychic upset from the loss, can result in an array of mental symptoms. Hypnogogic and hypnopompic hallucinations of the deceased person are normal occurrences in the days immediately following the loss of a spouse or sibling. Setting a place for the deceased at the dinner table or waiting for him to come home from work during this time is also not indicative of a pathological grief reaction.

It is crucial that both the griever and his family are told that this is a normal occurrence. This should allay their concerns and aid them through the important grieving process. Many cultures have clearly defined rituals which facilitate the working through of the grief. For example, a wake or professional wailers "allows" the person to express himself and "get it off of his chest," and removes the possibility of the individual seeing the expression of grief as a weakness or an embarrassment.

In the non-pathological or *normal grief reaction,* the working through requires acceptance of the loss, "giving up" the object and reconstituting the "void" that the loss has created. A failure to adequately resolve these conflicts means that the person will be left to operate from a state of intra-psychic dysequilibrium. This failure of resolution is one example of a pathological grief reaction.

The isolated and limited occurrence of symptoms such as hypnogogic hallucinations in the days following a loss does not require interventions such as neuroleptics or heavy sedation. It should be recalled that a short lived and isolated psychotic symptom does not constitute a functional psychosis anymore than a sharp pain radiating down the leg constitutes a herniated vertebral disc. Many of the symptoms discussed earlier as characteristic of a major affective disorder can occur in a normal grief reaction. It is likely that these symptoms will resolve themselves spontaneously within a week to ten days of normal grieving. Their appearance does not warrant the use of antidepressants but an hypnotic may have a place for a few days if insomnia becomes symptomatic.

Dysphoria is most likely the prominent symptom in a normal grief reaction. Depression, sadness and tears are to be expected. The person will display despondency and communicate a sense of being abandoned by the deceased. There may be features of anger, hostility and resentment which should be appropriately recognised and expressed by the grieving person. It is just as important to ventilate these features of anger and fear as it is those of sadness and depression.

It was mentioned earlier that grief reactions can involve inanimate objects such as desires, values and expectations. An individual may go through a grieving process after retirement from a job or upon the realization that he is not going to achieve a long held goal. The loss need not be of a "tangible" nature, the only requirement is that the person registers an intrapsychic "void" with the accompanying intrapsychic conflict.

The *pathological grief reactions* can be discussed in terms of *delay, duration,* and *distortion.* The delayed reaction is often characterised by the person being described by the family as a "tower of strength" during his period of loss. He does not grieve but rather regroups immediately by adopting a set of coping mechanisms which will later prove to be problematic. He may never adequately work through the loss and may continue to operate from an impaired position.

On the other hand, the working through of the loss may not begin for months or years. When it does finally occur it may not be recognised as such by the person. Indeed, the family may find the psychiatric symptoms puzzling since he was "such a tower of strength after the loss of his wife last year."

Grief reactions become pathological in terms of duration when they are incompletely resolved and the original difficulties "smolder on." It is said that "She never quite got over the loss of her husband." The result is that the person continues to operate from a disturbed state and the biases of this position profoundly and continuously alter the person's lifestyle. Attempts to reopen and rework the loss may fail, one reason being that it is more acutely traumatic than the chronic impairment. A therapeutic trial of medications such as antidepressants can aid the resolution of this form of pathological grief reaction if coupled with psychotherapy.

Grief reactions become pathological in terms of distortion because of the particular symptom that arise. Symptoms such as illusions, hallucinations, anxiety and depression are to be expected in many cases for a short period of time. However, some patients may develop a more complete set of symptoms constituting a brief reactive psychosis or a major affective illness such as a primary depressive disorder. Suicidal ideation may be such that rapid intervention is required in the form of somatic treatment. As in the case of postpartum psychoses, there has been a "straw that broke the camel's back." Obviously, in all pathological grief reactions, psychological and sociological intervention is required for the person and his family.

CHAPTER 13

THE ETIOLOGY OF MAJOR AFFECTIVE DISORDER

As with the schizophrenias, a question to be asked is whether a unitary etiology is to be expected for the major affective disorders. Also, taking sides in a "nature versus nurture" debate concerning the etiology of major affective disorders is as counterproductive as in the case of the schizophrenias.

BIOLOGICAL THEORIES

A number of toxic-organic disorders result in symptoms which are characteristic of the primary affective disorders. These comprise part of the secondary affective disorders and are of major importance in the diagnosis of affective illness.

Whether these toxic-organic factors approximate, unmask or create the characteristic symptoms de novo remains in question. It may well be that the dysphoric symptoms are a "pure" psychological response to the toxic-organic disorder but nevertheless even these "pure" psychological features need a biological "vehicle" for their symptomatic expression.

Head trauma can result in the symptom profiles found in primary affective disorders. There is an interpatient consistency in the *form* of these symptoms which can be taken as "independent" of the psycho-social factors. For example, the *content* and communication of insomnia will significantly vary from patient to patient depending on such factors as their education, socio-economic group and cultural background but the form of the symptom, namely poor sleep, is the same. Studies show that affective symptoms, of both the depressive and manic type, are more related to lesions involving the non-dominant hemisphere of the brain. The disinhibited, labile and impulsive qualities of cognition, affect and behaviour found in functional mania is closely mimiced in frontal lobe syndromes due to infections, degenerative processes and tumors.

The classic example of affective symptoms associated with cerebral infection is syphilis. In its tertiary stage, so-called General Paresis of the Insane (GPI), there is notable involvement of the frontal lobes and manic symptoms involving grandiose delusions and disinhibited behaviour is well documented.

Modern psychosurgery focuses on the anterior limbic system to alleviate symptoms of chronic and intractable depressive disorders. Limbic seizures are well documented as producing symptoms characteristic of primary affective disorders. In this regard, convulsive therapies (ECT) are effective treatments for both the manic and depressed phases of primary affective disorders. These points will be discussed in more detail in a later chapter.

The fact that demonstrably organic disorders can mimic the symptoms seen in primary affective disorders does not necessarily mean that these functional disorders have some, as yet unidentified, unitary organic etiology. However, it does stress that their appearance requires a careful assessment of the patients medical status before concluding that the altered mental state is of a functional etiology.

The endocrinopathies, specifically the thyroid and adrenal abnormalities, offer important insights into the biological aspects of affective disorders. Thyroid disorders, Cushing's syndrome and pituitary dysfunction can feature symptoms characteristic of the affective disorders. The alleviation of these endorcrinopathies can result in the removal of the affective symptoms.

Adrenal hormones, particularly cortisol, are involved in regulation of mood and behaviour. Both endogenous and exogenous cortisol is well recognised as producing changes in mood. Anxiety is the commonest dysphoria induced by this hormone and under certain conditions elation similar to mania as well as psychomotor retardation is reported. Prolonged use of exogenous steroids, typically in excess of 60 mg of prednisone per day, can result in affective syndromes and clinical presentations similar to the brief reactive psychosis.

Variation in the normal circadian secretion of endogenous cortisol has been noted in patients with primary depressive disorders. This alteration has been suggested as a biological marker for this type of depressive illness. The dexamethasone suppression test (DST) will be discussed in more detail later in the text.

The pituitary and hypothalmic factors which govern the thyroid and adrenal glands, such as thyroid stimulating hormone (TSH) and thyroid releasing hormone (TRH), have been reported as low. Releasing hormone (TRH), has been reported as low and relatively non-responsive in primary depressive illness. It has also been reported that endogenous, in contrast to neurotic, depressions have a suppressed adrenal response to the administration of methylamphetamine.

Amphetamines were discussed earlier in connection with the schizophrenias. It was mentioned that, depending on the dosage and duration of administration, these drugs could produce both manic and depressive syndromes. The proposal is that manic-like states are due to increased synthesis and release of biogenic amines due to the action of these analeptics. In the depressive states, usually after prolonged use of amphetamines, there is a proposed exhaustion of neurotransmitters resulting in a biogenic amine depletion state.

Rauwolfia serpentini compounds have been used for centuries in India as a tranquiliser in the treatment of "mental" disorders. In the western hemisphere, the rauwolfian derivitive reserpine has been used principally as an antihypertensive. Its mode of action can be summarised as the depletion of catecholamines and indolamines by promoting their release from presynaptic storage vesicles resulting in their exposure to degrading enzymes. These neutrotransmitters are therefore unavailable as sympathomimetic agents and one result will be a reduction of blood pressure. However, in addition there is a reduction in the availabilityy of these biogenic amines as mediators of mood. Therefore, in accordance with the biogenic amine hypothesis of major depressive disorders a likely complication of reserpine therapy for hypertension is the induction of a depressive syndrome. This is frequently seen in clinical practise when high doses are given in chronic treatment.

In passing, the dopamine hypothesis of schizophrenia proposes that this disorder is due to a relative "excess" of dopamine at the post-synapic terminal receptor. Therefore, reserpine might be effective in treatment of schizophrenia by depletion of the neurotransmitter pool. Indeed, in the 1950's, reserpine was used, with notable success, in the treatment of schizophrenia. Later, the neuroleptics via their post-synaptic receptor blockade proved to be more effective agents for the treatment of this functional psychosis.

Many patients with tuberculosis who were being treated with isoniazid showed distinct improvement in their overall mood. In some instances, previously depressed patients went on to develop manic symptoms whilst being treated with this agent. As a result a varient of this antituberculous drug, iproniazid, was developed as an antidepressant. This mode of action of iproniazid is the inhibition of monoamine oxidase (MAO) enzymes which are involved in the breakdown of catecholamines and indolamines as well as other biogenic amines. As would be expected, a problem was encountered in the treatment of some patients with these drugs is hypertension.

In simple terms, the implication is that drugs which "increase" biogenic amine neurotransmitter availability will have some effectiveness as antidepressants. The monoamine oxidase inhibitors (MAOI), such as iproniazid, perform this task by preventing neurotransmitter breakdown. A brief administration of an analeptic, such as amphetamine, increases synthesis and intersynaptic release of neurotransmitters as well as producing some inhibition of the degrading enzymes. This drug may offer "elevation" of mood but it is likely to be short lived and is not without risk regarding schizophrenic-like reactions.

The neurotransmitters are broken down primarily in the presynaptic terminal. This requires an active reuptake across the pre-synaptic terminal membrane for neurotransmitters located in the synaptic cleft. Therefore, a drug which blocks this active reuptake step would "increase" the availability of neurotransmitters within the synaptic cleft. This is the mode of action of the tricyclic antidepressants. As would be expected, these drugs have a structure similar to the neuroleptics since they also are required to "incorporate" in synaptic membranes.

Parkinsonian patients have a reduction of catecholamine synthesis in the substantia nigra. A method of treatment is to give L-dopa which is a precursor of the neurotransmitter dopamine. It was noted that some of these patients had a significant improvement in their mood whilst being on L-dopa for treatment of the movement disorder. This is in keeping with the previous points concerning the relationship of neurotransmitters and depressive disorders.

It is helpful in a discussion of the neurotransmitter hypothesis of the major affective disorders to refer to Figure 18 which is on page 87.

In its simplest terms, this hypothesis proposes that the depressive phase of a major affective disorder is due to a reduction of available neurotransmitters and the manic phase resulting from an excess. The point must be made that the neurotransmitter's role in major affective disorders may be as a "regulator" of the mood state rather than the "basic drive." That is to say, the symptoms may arise from a modulation effect by the disturbed biogenic amines on a multifactorial set of parameters which together define the persons basic mood.

Direct assay of the neurotransmitters, such as dopamine, norepinephrine and serotonin, is limited in human subjects other than in exceptional clinical cases. Hence, one has to approximate the situation by looking at neurotransmitter breakdown products which, as was mentioned earlier in connection with the dopamine hypothesis of schizophrenia, is at best a second hand method.

The *catecholamine hypothesis* focuses on norepinephreine's principle metabolite, 3-methyoxy-4-hydroxyphenylglycol (MHPG). Studies suggest that the urinary and cerebrospinal fluid levels of MHPG, as well as the levels of norepinephreine itself, are low in primary depressive disorders compared to the findings in secondary depressive illness. The low values are particularly found in bipolar depressed patients.

The tricyclic antidepressants and the newer "second generation" antidepressants, which will be discussed in more detail in a later chapter, block the active reuptake of norepinephrine at the presynaptic terminal membrane to varying degrees. It has been proposed that patients with symptoms of a primary depressive disorder and low levels of MHPG might show a better clinical response with antidepressants which have a relative preference for blockade of norepinephrine reuptake. It may be that patients with these symptoms who do not have a low MHPG level would do better on antidepressants which show a preference for serotonin reuptake blockade.

Along the same lines of choosing a particular antidepressant, it has been said the primary depressive patients who show a transient improvement in mood following a low dose challenge with amphetamine may respond better to predominantly norepinephrine blocking antidepressants. These points are well taken but should not be considered as "written in stone." Perhaps, as will be discussed later in more detail, a more crucial factor in the choice of medication is being able to ensure an adequate therapeutic trial of a drug in light of its relative side-effects and contraindications.

The *indolamine hypothesis* of primary depressive disorders focuses on serotonin and its principle metabolite 5-hydroxyindolacetic acid (5-HIAA). Studies find that in some depressed patients there is a reduction in the urine and cerebrospinal fluid levels of this metabolite. It has been reported that there is a higher risk of suicide and violence in primary depressive patients with decreased 5-HIAA levels.

The biogenic amine hypotheses suggest an increase of neurotransmitters and their metabolities in the manic phase of primary affective disorders. Recent studies show that manics had significantly elevated levels of MHPG in their cerebrospinal fluid compared to normal controls. Furthermore, the degree of elevation of MHPG follows the severity of the mania symptom rating score. The 5-HIAA levels in cerebrospinal fluid was not different in manic patients compared to normal controls. The changes in cerebrospinal MHPG levels were not reflected by raised MHPG levels in the manic's urine.

It was mentioned earlier that sleep disturbance is a characteristic feature of primary affective illness. In simple terms, the REM stages of sleep are mediated via catecholamines and the slow wave or non-REM stages are modulated through a serotinergic system. A feature of the sleep staging in primary depression is a reduction in REM latency with a decrease in non-REM Stage 3 and 4. Studies show a progressive recovery of Stage 3 and 4 and prolongation of REM latency as the primary depressive syndrome resolves. Perhaps antidepressants with a preference for serotinergic reuptake blockade would be more effective in major depression which features a sleep disturbance as one of its symptoms. It should be noted that some benzodiazepines have been reported as suppressing Stages 3 and 4.

If depressed subjects are sleep deprived for a number of days and then allowed to sleep, there is an excess or rebound effect of Stages 3 and 4 in the early sleep recovery. This rebound phenomena can be viewed as an attempt at compensation. Therefore, sleep depriving a patient with a primary depression for a few days and then allowing him uninterrupted sleep may produce the same Stage 3 and 4 recovery as the antidepressants. However, the sleep deprived rebound phenomena is, unlike the antidepressant induced recovery of these stages, short lived. Furthermore, sleep deprivation would likely add other symptoms to the depressive profile which would be problematic.

In neuronal transmission, the so-called sodium pump plays a crucial role and catecholamines are known to influence its activity. In primary depression, studies suggest that there is a decrease in sodium pump activity which increases the intracellular retention of sodium. This is consistent with other neurophysiological findings in primary depression such as decreased arousal thresholds and increased average evoked potentials. This interface of the neurotransmitter hypothesis and membrane transport is interesting in view of the effectiveness of lithium in the treatment of a number of phases of primary affective disorders.

As in the case of the biological theories of schizophrenia, the biological hypotheses of the major affective disorders are tantalising and provocative. The paralleled development of psychopharmacology with neurophysiology and neurochemistry has been revolutional in the field of psychiatry. In attempting to formulate a biological etiology for neuropsychiatric disorders, the complexity of the problem must be always borne in mind.

PSYCHOLOGICAL THEORIES

The word *depression* can refer to a clinical syndrome, such as a primary or secondary affective disorder, and a symptom in the sense of sad, unhappy or "blue." Furthermore, the word depression may be used by a patient to communicate problems of cognition, perception, mobility and behaviour as well as affect and mood. This is to be expected given the interdependence of the components which make up the composite mental state. The complaint of depression is so ubiquitous in life and clinical practise that taken in isolation it is often meaningless and frequently misleading.

The symptom and syndromes of depression indicate a perturbation within the mental state. The critical issue concerns the degree of associated pathology and its etiology. Earlier in the text, the "need versus fear" model concerning the creation of mental symptoms was discussed. Briefly, this proposed that symptoms developed because they helped to restore intrapsychic equilibrium. This model can be applied to certain aspects of the depressive syndrome.

For example, depressive symptomatology in bereavement has a protective role during this period of turmoil and helps facilitate the necessary grieving process. In fact, the absence of a depressive reaction in bereavement may be more ominous than its occurrence. A secondary depressive disorder, for example in connection with an adjustment reaction or a life threatening illness, can be viewed as "having certain advantages." The depressive feature may facilitate both a psychological and physiological" withdrawal from an intolerable situation" as well as "draw attention to the turmoil." This should not be taken to mean that the development of depressive features indicates a deliberateness or manipulation by the grieving individual. Also, the process is not without much "pain." It may well be that the ability to experience and express depression is a "built in safeguard" in the manner that experiencing anxiety has "warning" properties which aid in survival.

Some points concerning psychoanalytic theory were discussed earlier in reference to the psychological theories of schizophrenia. The libidinal, topographic and structural models of the mind were outlines and some key terms were defined. This information will be used in the following discussion of the psychological aspects of depression and mania.

A concept which is central to the psychological theories of depression is that the individual experiences a *loss of self-esteem*. An individual's self-esteem is, according to psychoanalytic theory, a function, in part, of their psychosexual development. Similarly what the individual takes to be a loss of self-esteem and the nature of the coping mechanisms employed as a result will be dependent on psychosexual maturation. The concept of self-esteem involves numerous factors such as the acquired ego functions, self-worth, integrity, values, role and object relations.

Psychoanalytic theory stresses the importance of developmental processes which occur during early childhood. During this critical development period, important mental substrates are laid down which will have a great influence on later stages of maturation and development. Since psychosexual maturation is an ongoing process, an individual's self-esteem is constantly being redefined and integrated, as well as traumatised, throughout the life cycle.

A loss of self-esteem is a traumatisation which results in some degree of intrapsychic conflict. The immediate coping response is a *regression* by some aspects of mental function in order to re-establish some intrapsychic equilibrium. By definition, regressive means that there will be a re-emergence of mental functions which are characteristic of an earlier form of mental function. Although regression brings about a temporary solution it "weakens" the mental state by virtue of the relative primitiveness of its functions.

An important component of self-esteem is object relations. As was pointed out earlier, their representation will depend on the degree of psychosexual development. Regression involving the object relations means that they will be of a more primitive type of representation.

In depressive disorders, the psychoanalytic theories propose that regression takes place to the oral and anal stages of psychosexual development because it is at this early stage of development that the person had "flaws" in their maturation process. Object relations at these early stages are characteristically *ambivalent* in their representation. They are not in the form of a mature single composite representation but rather consist of two antithetical components which can mutually coexist in the primitive mental stage.

As a paradigm for depression, one can consider a loss associated with bereavement. A particular example is the situation relating to the death of a spouse. Firstly, we can consider the psychoanalytic "steps" of *normal grief* associated with this type of loss. This is schematically shown in the following figure.

The loss creates a "void" within the mental state which gives rise to an instability, namely intrapsychic dysequilibrium. The immediate response is some regression in an attempt to counteract the results of the loss. This causes a distortion of the ego boundary (Figure 34c). Therefore, as a

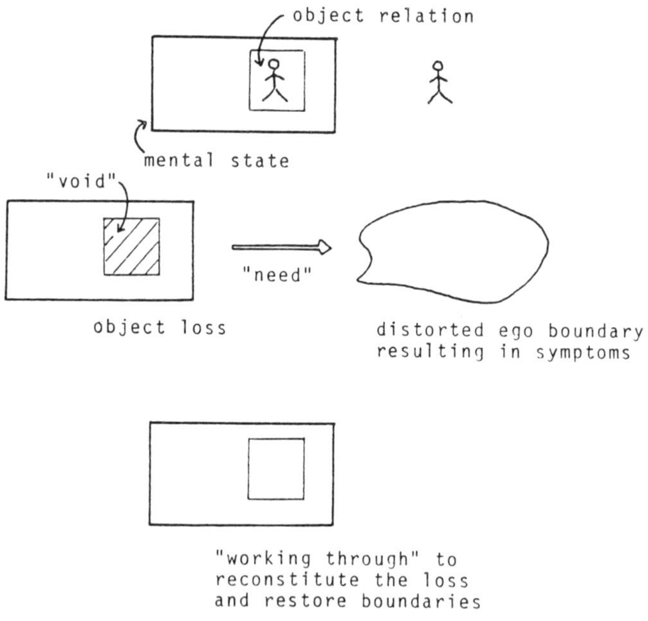

Figure 34

consequence of the regression in a normal grief reaction, symptoms will arise which reflect this ego boundary distortion. This may include illusions, hallucinations, dysphoria and paranoid ideation. The symptoms are the "price paid" for the needed regression in order to deal with the fear created by the loss.

The working through of this normal grief reaction involves the redefining of the mental sets, particularly those involving the mental representation of the object loss. This working through and resolution of the grief will reconstitute the "void" and eliminate the need for the ego boundary distortion. When this has been successfully completed, there will be no "need" for the symptoms such as hallucinations and dysphoria. The symptoms provide a temporary stabilising measure in the face of the intrapsychic turmoil.

A *pathological grief reaction* does not follow the above steps and it offers a *depressive paradigm.* During the early stages of psychosexual development, the theory proposes that incomplete resolution of intrapsychic stresses occur which produce "flaws" in aspects of the overall mental maturation. These "flaws" are points to which a part of mental functioning is likely to regress if the individual is subjected to a critical intrapsychic stress in later years. This propensity of early psychosexual trauma to produce "flaws" which can later manifest as an adult mental disorder is approximated by the phrase "the child is father to the man."

The classical psychoanalytic concept is that individuals predisposed to depression reactions, such as pathological grief reactions, have encountered difficulties with object relations during the oral-anal phase of psychosexual development. For example, they have suffered significant losses, such as the death of a parent, at these early stages of development. The associated "flaws" may "lay dormant" as the general mental development continues but their presence will influence subsequent maturation to some degree and may severe as a critical point of regression under later intrapsychic stress.

The parental loss need not be in the obvious form of a death. It could be an equivalence of the parent being "lost" in terms of the child's primitive mental functioning. Inconsistencies in the parent-child interaction could be interpreted as such losses by the child and result in tenuous object relations being formed, a poor self-image and a lack of basic trust.

In a pathological grief reaction, the steps to work through and "give up" the lost object are not set in motion. Instead, regression takes place such that particular coping mechanisms characteristic of the oral-anal phase come into operation to re-establish intrapsychic equilibrium. The defence mechanism employed, which is characteristic of this phase of development, is *incorporation.* The lost object is retained by this act of *internalisation* and the "void" is pathologically reconstituted. Since the retaining is by a primitive mechanism then the mental representation of the internalised object will be primitive. The internalised object will have *ambivalent* representation within the mental state. This is schematically shown in the following figure.

The spouse is incorporated in the form of a "good" and a "bad" object. These antithetical representations coexist within the mental state. Feelings of anger, hostility and guilt which were previously directed towards the spouse are now, because of internalisation, directed "against the self." The eliminating or destruction of the "bad" object can result in suicidal ideation and acts.

The greater the regression in response to the intrapsychic trauma of the loss then the greater will be the primitiveness and the more ambivalent will be the representation of the introjected object. Therefore, the greater will be the primitive "bad" internalised object and so the greater is the risk of suicide associated with this pathological grief reaction.

In the layman's sense, the word ambivalent is frequently used to signify indecision, vascillation and mixed feelings. In such a case, the ambivalent object is still a single com-

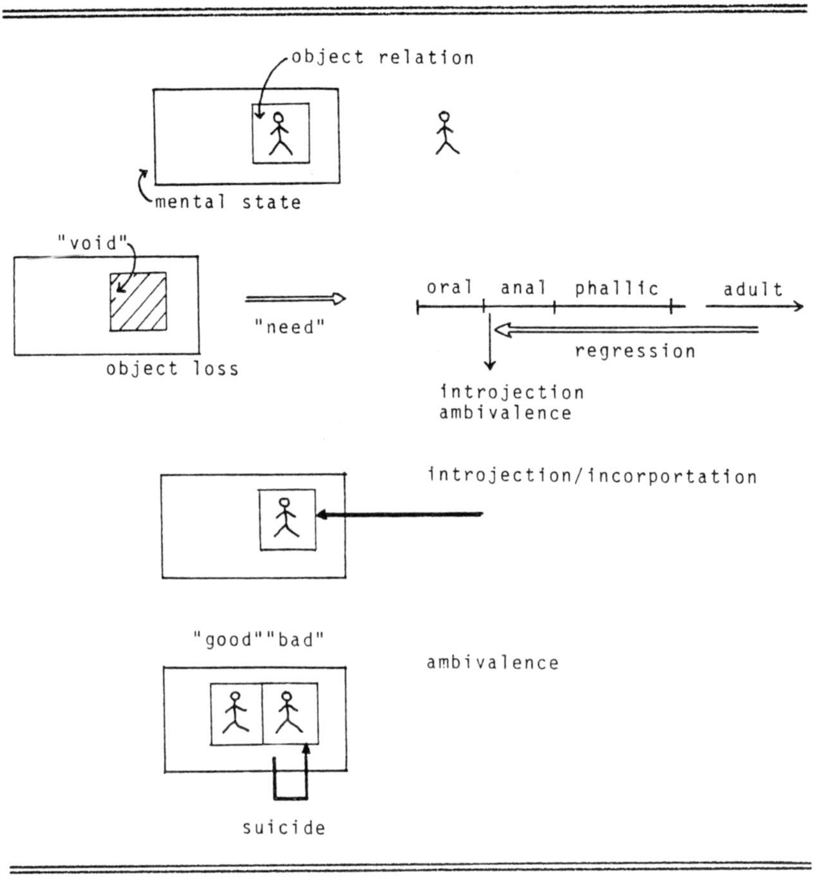

Figure 35

posite object though with two "opposite" portions. It would follow that in this sense the greater the ambivalence then the less likely would be the risk of suicide due to the indecisiveness or vascillation. This point illustrates the need to use terms such as ambivalence correctly when discussing the depressive paradigm.

Problems relating to loss and abandonment can be further illustrated by considering the case of a young child being hospitalised, for example, for a tonsillectomy. The child's notion and understanding of what is happening and why is based on immature and relatively primitive mental processes. There is no point discussing the situation in terms of recurrent abcesses, surgery or the medical model. It should not be too surprising if the child "sees" the situation as "ripping my throat because I kept stealing ice cream from my kid sister."

For this young child, the object relations involving parents, his basic trust, self worth and self-esteem are primitive and, perhaps more importantly, "brittle." The notions of time are also immature so that a separation due to hospitalisation lasting days may be processed as equivalent to months on an adult scale. Therefore, a short separation from "weakly" held objects can have the impact of total abandonment with devastating results.

The parents going home and leaving this child "at a loss" may result in him experiencing a pathological grief reaction. Initially, the child will likely be angry and "protest" the perceived abandonment. Attempts made to console and reassure the child by the hospital staff will likely be unsuccessful. A few days later, the child is reported as "improving, less upset, more settled, coming around and warming up to the nurses and staff." In the terms of a grief reaction, there has been a working through and giving up of parental object relations. The void has been reconstituted by objects "found" on the ward. When, some time later, the parents return they may be rejected and shunned by the child. The steps will probably reoccur when the child is now "abandoned" by the hospital introjects and returns home with his parents.

It is likely that multiple hospitalisations in early childhood increases the development of impaired object relations. Those object relations involving the parents would be particularly critical. The linking of such impairments of the developing mind to the risk of developing adult depressive disorders can be discussed with reference to the superego.

The superego is formed during the resolution of the oedipal conflict which occurs towards the end of the phallic stage of psychosexual development. This unit of the mind can be viewed as a set of internal sanctions, an important component of which involves the introjection of parental images. The superego is intimately involved with the formation and expression of basic trust, ego ideals and strengths as well as the important concept of self-esteem.

Therefore, introjection of 'distorted" parental images in early childhood will result in altered superego function and concepts of self-esteem. For example, if the parental introjects during early critical stages are "archaic and punative" then the subsequent superego ideals and sanctions will be "harsh, unattainably demanding and hypercritical." This increases the risk of failing to "satisfy the superego's expectations" making traumatic losses in self-esteem and development of depressive disorders more likely.

An obvious example, as mentioned earlier, of such a distortion is the infant's perceived abandonment by the parent in the formative years. The ultimate abandonment would be the parent's death at this point in the child's life. However, study of patients who suicided due to a major depressive disorder failed to demonstrate that they had a higher occurrence of the death of a parent during the patient's childhood compared to a control group. Nevertheless, as mentioned earlier, an infant's primitive mental processes may perceive that the parent is "gone for good" due to events other than actual death of the parent.

The normal "arrangement" of the three components of the Structural Theory has the superego aligned with the ego so that its sanctions can aid in the ego's containment of but utilisation of the id. Mania can be discussed in terms of a pathological shift in this alignment such that the superego now "joins with" the id rather than the ego. The necessary containment of the id by the ego is thereby critically lessened and weakened resulting in a more "unbridled" and pathological id expression. The result can be the symptoms characteristic of mania such as impulsivity, lack of judgement and restraint, grandiosity and poorly controlled demands for instant gratification indicating the reduction in sanctions.

In one sense, mania can be viewed as a defence against depression. Mania following a depressive state could be viewed as a flight into health. It was noted earlier that there is a similarity in the form of symptoms found in mania and depression. In terms of this theory one notes that the elevated sense of self-esteem of mania has a brittleness, vulnerability and self-destructive quality akin to that associated with the reduced self-esteem seen in depression. It has been said that "scratch a manic and you will find a depressive."

Though there is a continual reworking and development of intrapsychic processes throughout life, classical psychoanalytic theory stresses the importance of the early phases of this process. If early defects occur, the individual continues to operating from a potentially *dysthymic position* and is likely prone to continuing problems of mood disturbances throughout life both of a primary and secondary nature.

SOCIOLOGICAL THEORIES

As with any other illness, the affecive disorders are neither developed or experienced in a vacuum. Dysphoria, like it or not, is ubiquitous and colours everyone's lifestyle to varying degrees of severity.

If everyone with a dysphoria was identified in a given catchment area at a particular time, it is more than likely that the majority of the dysphorias would be in response to some psycho-social stress and not be related to primary affective disorders. Most of these dysphorias would spontaneously recover and be considered by those involved as simple "life." Others would require hospitalisation. However, all of these disorders are complicated to some degree by sociological factors. Even if these factors are secondary, they are crucial in the overall outcome of the dysphoria.

Theories concerning the family and social dynamics of affective disorders are intimately coupled to the psychological theories. Interactions within a family provides a vehicle for developing as well as coping with intrapsychic conflict and the characteristics and learnt behaviours operating within a family constellation will colour the clinical presentation of an affective syndrome. The expression and emphasis of the disorder and its subsequent outcome will be greatly influenced by social factors. This is true for all medical illness.

The sociological scheme may allow a primary affective disorder to "smolder" unrecognised and untreated for long periods if not forever. The social "stigma" associated with mental illness often prevents a patient seeking or receiving appropriate treatment. There is no doubt that many patients are self critical because of such stigma and their family's misunderstanding of the disorders adds to the difficulties instituting treatment. Statements such as "Thank God it's a brain tumor and not something wrong with his head" are far from rare. One would do well to compare the treatment successes of brain tumors to that of major affective disorders.

It is true that all affective illnesses feature sociological stresses. However, it does not necessarily follow that these sociological stresses are etiological. Furthermore, the fact that there is a clinical response to social intervention does not prove that the social factors are the sole etiology. If patients with a primary affective illness have evidence of family chaos one must ask whether this is a cause or a response to the affective disorder.

The crucial point is that affective illnesses must be approached from the triple viewpoint of biological, psychological and sociological theories. Evenso one notes the additional fact that the "treated" patient who returns to continuing social chaos is likely to relapse to some degree.

CHAPTER 14

STATISTICS AND GENETICS OF MAJOR AFFECTIVE DISORDERS

It has been said that the major affective disorders constitute the most mistreated of major medical illnesses. The misidentification of these disorders, in the form of false positive and false negative diagnosis, is very frequent. Since these disorders are "malignant," affecting both the patient and his associates, this point is most unfortunate particularly since modern treatment is very successful in the majority of cases.

Information concerning genetics and statistics of these disorders is helpful in focusing on the diagnosis and offer a perspective in planning health care delivery. There is an age of risk for the development of the major affective disorders ranging from 15 to 60 years of age. It is rare for the primary affective disorders to present before the age of 15 years and presentation prior to the onset of puberty is questionable. Cases having their first presentation after 60 years of age do occur but it is likely that many of these have been present for some time in an unrecognised form.

For women, the risk of presenting with a primary affective disorder peaks during the child-bearing years and points to the importance of screening for postpartum disorders. In any given year, some 15 percent of people between 15 and 60 years of age will present with a major affective disorder. It is said that less than 5 percent of these will receive adequate treatment. However, some 10 percent of prescriptions, both new and refills, are for the treatment of "depression." One has to wonder how many of these prescriptions are to treat the disorder and how many are given because of the isolated symptom of depression. Also, one wonders how many were for a homeopathic dose of medication and how many are for medications, such as anxiolytics, which have no primary value in the treatment of major depressive syndromes.

It must be borne in mind that suicide is a significant problem associated with the major affective disorders. In the bipolar disorders, one percent will commit suicide within six months of being identified. The rate of suicide for patients with a primary affective disorder over their lifetime is some 15 percent. Taken as a whole, the major affective disorders have a suicide rate of 0.5 percent. The difference in lethality of the primary affective disorders compared to the general affective disorders should be noted.

Perhaps only a few percent of major affective disorder patients are hospitalised. Nevertheless, patients with a diagnosis of depression constitute some 30 percent of patients admitted to the psychiatric units of general hospitals. If one considers the mental hospitals, as opposed to general hospital psychiatric units, 14 males and 28 females per one hundred thousand population are admitted per year with a diagnosis of a major affective disorder (Table 1).

A few years ago, it was noted that in the United Kingdom many more patients were hospitalised with a diagnosis of bipolar disorder than in the United States. The diagnosis was some 18 times commoner in the United Kingdom. A significant, and perhaps major reason, was the tendency in the United States to diagnose patients with symptoms such as formal thought disorders, delusions and hallucinations of functional etiology as schizophrenic. The study illustrating this so-called "schizomania" for the diagnosis of schizophrenia in the United States showed a much greater diagnostic agreement between United Kingdom clinicians than between their American counterparts. It was said that the lower agreement between U.S. clinicians regards diagnosis reflected their greater use of psychodynamic and interperative approaches compared to their British counterparts.

The problems associated with determinations of incidence and prevalence for the schizophrenias was discussed in an earlier chapter. The nature of affecive disorders suggests that these problems will be perhaps even more apparent, however, there is a consistency of results from the various studies.

The prevalence of major affective disorders has been estimated as high as 2 per 100 population, a factor ten times as great as for the schizophrenias. The "cost" of the major affective disorders in terms of productivity or dollars and cents can only be guessed.

The lifetime expectancy or risk of morbidity over a person's lifespan for schizophrenia was approximately 1 percent and equal in males and females. In the case of bipolar disorders, the morbidity risk in males is some 2.0 percent and 3.0 percent in females. This lifetime expectancy dramatically increases if the person has a positive family history of major affective disorders, particularly of the bipolar type.

The epidemiological data stresses the need to distinguish the bipolar and unipolar disorders from the overall major affective illnesses. The primary affective disorders show a characteristic age of risk, symptom profile, lack of necessary and sufficient precipitants and genetic loading. For a given identified patient, the so-called index case, the risk of his sibling manifesting a primary affective disorder during their lifetime is markedly increased to some 12 percent. If the index case has a parent with a primary affective disorder, then the sibling risk increases to some 25 percent.

In the general population, the risk of having an alcoholic father is some 2 percent but when coupled with a primary affective disorder the chance increases five fold. If the index case for a primary affective disorder has a parent manifesting this disorder along with alcoholism, then the risk of a sibling having a primary affective illness during their lifetime increases to some 50 percent.

As was the case in schizophrenia, the expectancy of an index case's family member manifesting a primary affective disorder decreases as the relationship to the index case "weakens." The data for schizophrenia was given in Table 2 and that for primary affective disorders is summarised below.

```
Negative Family History

lifetime risk of becoming an index case with
a bipolar disorder is 2% for males and some
3% for females

Positive Family History

index case's sibling's lifetime risk 12%
index case's child's lifetime risk 8%
index case's parent's lifetime risk 5%
index case's uncle/stepsibling's risk 2%
```

Table 3 (b)

Studies have shown that the bipolar and unipolar disorders have different family loadings reflected by a positive family history. The family loading for the bipolar is some 15 times stronger than the unipolar. Additional information can be obtained from the concordance rates in twin studies, for example, rates of concordance for monozygotic and dizygotic twins differ for the bipolar and unipolar disorders. Although these studies are difficult to carry out for a number of reasons, the information has a consistency which is outlined in the following table.

The primary affective disorders and nuclear schizophrenias do not "cross load" for one another. That is to say, a positive family history for schizophrenia increases the expectancy of schizophrenia for members of that family but does not increase the risk for primary affective disorders. A positive family history for primary affective disorders "loads" other family members for these disorders but not for the nuclear schizophrenias.

Twin Study Concordance Rates

Manic-depressive (Kallman)	monozygotic twins	100%	
	dizygotic twins	25%	
Other studies	bipolar disorders	85%	monozygotic
	unipolar disorders	25%	monozygotic
	bipolar disorders	40%	dizygotic
	unipolar disorders	25%	dizygotic

Table 4

The major depressive syndrome of involutional melancholia is interesting in terms of a "cross load." The overall expectation of nuclear schizophrenia in the family of a person suffering from involutional melancholia is some 6 percent. This is approximately 6 fold the risk of schizophrenia manifesting in a person who has a negative family history for nuclear schizophrenia. Some of the symptoms characteristic of involutional melancholia, such as primary delusions and Schneiderian first rank symptoms, suggest a "cross over" with the nuclear schizophrenias and may account for this apparant loading.

It was pointed out earlier that symptoms which are characteristic of affective disorders are common in the presentation of the atypical schizophrenias. In some atypical schizophrenias, a positive family history of major functional disorders is for affective disorders rather than for nuclear schizophrenias. Probably, the atypical psychosis which is most suggestive of this "cross over" is the schizo-affective subtype. It is well to consider that the functional psychoses lie on a spectrum rather than at two isolated poles.

When the genetic studies are critically reviewed in terms of the rigor of inclusion criteria, study design and application, there is ample evidence of the primary affective disorders having a genetic transmission. The indications are of a single and dominant gene with variable penetrance. This is in contrast to the polygenetic recessive transmission with variable penetrance for the nuclear schizophrenias.

The question in terms of the primary affective disorders is whether this dominant gene is autosomal or sex linked. The fact that the morbidity risk is approximately twice as high in females as in males suggests an X-linked factor. However, if it is X-linked and dominant then transmission from father to son would be classically excluded. However, such an inheritance pathway is seen in clinical practise. An autosomal linkage would avoid this particular problem but would not account for the preponderance of the primary affective disorders in females.

A number of elegant studies of bipolar patients and their families suggests that the bipolar disorder is an X-linked inheritance. It was found that in these families the female members were affected twice as often as males and maternal relatives twice as often as paternal relatives. It was also found in some of these studies of bipolar families that expression of the bipolar disorder was associated with the expression of colour blindness which was of an X-linked type. Also, the expression of bipolar disorders was found in association with the Xg blood group which is a genetic marker on the X chromosome.

CHAPTER 15

TREATMENT OF THE MAJOR AFFECTIVE DISORDERS

These disorders can be treated but not cured. The treatment of any clinical disorder, whether schizophrenia, a major affective disorder or a broken hip, should be approached under the headings of biological, psychological and sociological. The presentation of the clinical syndromes of the major affective disorders makes it often very difficult to identify the necessary blending of these three approaches to produce the maximum beneficial response. Nevertheless, it is crucial to approach cases from this triple viewpoint.

SOCIOLOGICAL TREATMENT

A critical issue in the treatment of major affective disorders is that the patient, their family, and in many instances their clinician, recognize that these disorders are illnesses akin to such as hypertension, diabetes mellitus and so on. It should be made clear to the patient and others that the appropriate treatment may have a better overall success than the treatment of many other medical disorders.

If the major affective disorders are viewed as weakness, lack of effort or, and this is not an exaggeration, a "sin" then the results can be tragic. The stigma of shame and embarrassment which so often accompanies these disorders can result in the problem being "swept under the carpet" and ignored.

The social disruption which can preceed, accompany and result from a major affective disorder should not be allowed to compound. Furthermore, it must be dealt with in order to maximize the patient's recovery. Despite alleviation of the rank symptoms of a major affective disorder, the social problems may still sabotage the overall recovery. It is important that ground work of a supportive and insightful nature is begun with the patient's family and associates when the patient is hospitalized. If the patient is discharged without this having been initiated, there is a great likelihood of a relapse. As a comparison, one must work with the families of a diabetic patient before discharging the patient from the hospital.

The role of the social worker cannot be overemphasized. Their information is helpful in formulating the problem and invaluable in designing a comprehensive treatment plan.

PSYCHOLOGICAL TREATMENT

The nature of major affective disorders makes it obvious that psychological treatment is important in all major affective disorders. For many major affective disorders psychotherapy is the mainstay of treatment. In many of these cases, the biological modes of treatment, such as pharmacotherapy, have little value and in some instances, are counter productive. One must prevent a patient relying totally on a "magic pill."

All too often, clinicians "reach for the pad" and prescribe some medication which is neither indicated or sufficient. It is ludicrous to think that a secondary affective disorder due to marital strife will resolve if one, or both, of the partners "take a pill." It should be borne in mind that the medication may be used to "blot out the issues" and avoid dealing with problems and may be taken as a sign of ascribing responsibility to a particular person for all of the problems.

The issue is not whether psychotherapy is indicated in the treatment of a major affective disorder but rather which type of psychotherapy will be the most effective in a particular case. There are many forms of psychological therapy, for example, psychoanalysis, psychoanalytic psychotherapy and "general" psychotherapy. In a given patient, it may be best in the form of individual or group therapy and it can vary in terms of appropriate directiveness and focus.

The details of the various psychological therapies are beyond the scope of this text but some general points can be made. A proposition of psychoanalysis is that abnormalities have occurred in the person's early psychosexual development and are now manifesting in the adult as the major affective illness. It is necessary to identify these abnormalities and rework the associated issues to reconstruct the intrapsychic processes thereby eliminating the need for the symptoms. Invariably, this is both a long and costly undertaking. Psychoanalysis cannot be used in many cases of major affective disorders and in some is clearly a professional error.

In psychoanalytic psychotherapy, the psychoanalytic principles are applied in a less "rigid" manner. There is a greater degree of directiveness on the part of the therapist with more emphasis on insight and alternative employment of the patients available intrapsychic processes to cope. There is less focus on the "there and then" of early psychosexual development and more on the "here and now" of recent problems. The group psychotherapy process offers support and identification as an augmentation of the individual treatment process.

BIOLOGICAL TREATMENT

The principle biological or somatic therapies are electroconvulsive therapy (ECT), lithium and antidepressants. The latter can be divided into tricyclics, monoamine oxidase inhibitors and the so-called "second generation" drugs.

1. Electroconvulsive Therapy (ECT)

This is one of the most misused and misunderstood treatments in psychiatry. It is often used in the treatment of disorders for which it has no established benefit. The misunderstandings of the treatment has led to its acquiring a 'reputation" which is unfounded.

Prior to the availability of controlled seizures as a treatment for the functional psychoses, the prognosis for patients with these disorders was poor. Hospitalization, for the majority of patients, was essentially custodial in nature. In many instances, this was in facilities which were not "well funded." It was said that the majority of these patients had only a ten percent chance of being institutionalized for less than two years. During this time, there was a high risk of developing a so-called institutional syndrome which made a successful return to the community very unlikely.

The introduction of controlled seizures as a treatment for the functional psychoses is generally credited to von Meduna. He noted that generalised epilepsy was a rare condition in patients with a functional psychosis. The inference was that these two conditions were antagonistic to each other and therefore induction of generalised convulsions in patients with a functional psychosis might elleviate the symptoms of the psychosis.

This somatic therapy was introduced in the early 1900's and proved to be remarkable successful. Some 20 percent of schizophrenic patients and 40 percent of patients with a major affective disorders given this treatment showed marked improvement. If compared to the improvement seen with non-somatic therapies, these results were very impressive.

At this point, it is instructive to make some comments on epileptic seizures and convulsive disorders. Firstly, seizure thresholds are a necessary property of the central nervous system and the ability to convulse is an inherent characteristic. The clinical issue is not whether a patient has seizures but rather why this occurs and the possible ramifications of the convulsions having taken place.

Overall, the commonest cause of seizures is probably still idiopathic though there are many identifiable disorders which will induce the necessary neuronal "instability" to cause a seizure. For example, a primary lesion within the central nervous system such as a hemorrhage or a brain tumor can be the etiology and these problems must be rectified in order to prevent further seizures. Secondary pathology can alter the seizure threshold, for instance, endocrinopathies involving the thyroid and glucose levels, changes in the cerebral blood flow which disturbs the brain's supply of oxygen, and the effects of numerous drugs such as anesthetics and alcohol.

In the majority of instances listed above, it is not sufficient to prescribe an anticonvulsant, rather one has to identify the abnormality and correct the problem. For instance, prolonged hypoglycemia will rapidly result in central nervous system damage and the convulsions will simply be a reflection of this parenchymal insult. The major clinical concern is not the convulsions but rather the correcting of the underlying abnormality and its possible ramifications to the central nervous system.

Generalised seizures have additional sequelae once the convulsion begins such as sustained hypoxia during the intra-ictal phase or falling down stairs during a convulsion and breaking ones neck. As will be seen in the following discussion, there is no primary underlying pathology to cause problems in association with induced ECT and since it is given in a clinically controlled setting the seizure sequelae complications will also not arise.

There is a notion, held by many layman and clinicians alike, that 'ECT burns the brain." In order to put this point in some perspective consider the following example. If a medical student has three generalized convulsions following an accident while playing football, one would not jump to the conclusion that he has suffered brain damage which will terminate his career. Assuming that he has no sequeale such as prolonged hypoxia, intracranial hemmorrhage, post traumatic subdural hematoma or fractured skull, then the issue of the post-epileptic brain damage would not be raised. Why, then, should this point be raised in connection with ECT?

Perhaps a major source of anxiety involving ECT is a question of "cosmetics." However, as will be discussed, patients do not "arch and thrash around" during ECT. Most people are disturbed by witnessing a generalized seizure and much of the anxiety is related to their sense of helplessness as the person convulses. Epilepsy involves that mysterious thing called the mind and, therefore, is surrounded by stigma, myths and plain ignorance.

An early mode of inducing a generalized tonic-clonic seizure in the treatment of functional psychoses involved the drug metrazol. Later, the gas, indoklon, was used for the controlled induction of a convulsion. In the 1930's, Cerletti devised an electrical method for seizure induction.

It must be noted that the effectiveness of generalized seizures in treating certain functional psychoses does not depend on the mode of induction of the convulsion. Drugs, gas and electricity are not significantly different in terms of therapeutic effectiveness. Electricity plays no part in the treatment other than inducing the generalized tonic-clonic seizure.

When ECT was first introduced as a treatment, the majority of patients were not given a general anesthetic for the procedure. This was not because "being aware of the procedure" was part of the therapy. The reason for no anesthesia, so-called *unmodified* ECT, was simply a matter of finance since the funds available for the care and treatment of mental patients at this time were pitifully lacking. Unmodified ECT is rarely, if ever, used today.

It is crucial that the patient receiving ECT is suffering from a disorder for which the treatment has been objectively shown to be effective. The correct diagnosis is the first step in the use of ECT. Controlled studies consistently show that it is effective in the treatment of both the manic and depressed phases of primary affective disorders. They report significant improvement in patients with primary depressive disorders in 70 to 80 percent of cases. Placebo treatments were effective, to some degree, in some 40 percent of cases indicating the marked superiority of ECT (it should be noted that ECT is not simply twice as effective as placebo). In general, ECT was slightly superior to antidepressant drugs in these controlled studies but it is not clear whether all of the patients receiving antidepressants were given adequate therapeutic trials of the medications.

The controlled studies did not indicate that ECT was useful in the treatment of secondary depressive disorders such a depressive neuroses, adjustment reactions with depressive symptoms and the psychoneuroses with depressive features. In many of these disorders, ECT was notably less successful than medications and placebo. This stresses the importance of correctly diagnosing the major affective disorders. A great deal of the controversial reputation of ECT is due to its application in disorders for which it is not indicated.

ECT is therapeutic for the manic phase of a bipolar disorder as on the depressive phase. The treatment of choice for an acute manic episode is lithium, perhaps initially with the addition of neuroleptics, but there are refractory cases of mania which require ECT. The studies suggest that if ECT is required to treat a manic episode, then more treatments will be required than for the alleviation of a depressive episode and they may have to be given twice per day. The average number of ECT treatments for a depressive episode is 7 or 8, depending on the studies.

The use of ECT in the treatment of schizophrenia is quite controversial. However, recent critical studies show that ECT is indicated in only one of the nuclear schizophrenias, namely, catatonic schizophrenia. There is great doubt as to its usefulness in hebephrenic and paranoid schizophrenia and a clear consensus that it is of little to no value in chronic schizophrenia. There is increasing evidence of ECT's usefulness in the atypical or non-nuclear schizophrenias. This might be expected given the "cross over" of symptomatology seen in the atypical schizophrenias, that is to say the brief reactive psychoses and schizophreniform disorders, and the primary affective disorders. The fact that many of the atypical schizophrenias turn out, after more history and information is collected, to be affective disorders may explain a portion of the "success" of ECT in these conditions.

There is no place for the use of ECT in the treatment of the classical neuroses or personality disorders. Likewise, it has no role in the treatment of chronic organic brain syndromes. However, it may well be that a geriatric patient has an organic brain syndrome plus a primary depressive disorder, in which case ECT may result in a significant overall improvement in the patient's mental functioning. In many of these cases ECT is preferable to the use of antidepressants since the latter have a number of relative contraindications which are not applicable to ECT.

Assuming that a given patient is suffering from one of the disorders for which ECT is indicated, then there are three points which suggest the use of ECT in preference to psychotropic medications and psychotherapy. These are *urgency, the failure of other treatments* and the *relative contraindications* of the other modes of treatment.

The disorders under consideration, such as primary depression and functional catatonia, have considerable morbidity and lethality. In some cases, this is to a degree requiring immediate clinical intervention. Frequently, medications and psychotherapy are unable to reduce the symptoms with the rapidity warranted by the clinical picture. For example, a pregnant woman with active suicidal intent due to an underlying primary depressive disorder requires symptom relief in days, not weeks or months. Furthermore, there is a potentially "double" lethality in such a case.

Studies show that ECT begins to reverse the symptoms characteristic of primary depression sooner than antidepressants or psychotherapy. The same is true for agitated or retarded functional catatonia which, because of numerous secondary complications, particularly in the elderly, has notable morbidity and mortality.

Even one-to-one observation of a patient does not guarantee against suicide attempts or successes. More importantly, one-to-one involvement need not, in fact often will not, significantly reduce the patient's anxiety and turmoil. This sustained anxiety could seriously harm, for example, a pregnant woman's unborn child.

The second indication for the use of ECT involves the relative contraindications for psychotherapy and psychotropics in some cases. In terms of psychotherapy, many clinical presentations simply rule out this form of treatment to any significant degree. Also, psychotherapy has not been shown to be effective in influencing the first rank symptoms of the functional psychoses. The simple fact is that psychotherapy is of little value in the case of a mute and immobile catatonic or a grossly psychotic and suicidal patient. Psychotropic medications have a range of side effects and relative contraindications which may prevent their use in some cases. Those associated with neuroleptics were discussed in detail in an earlier section and a number of these side effects occur with the antidepressants medications. Specific problems relating to these medications arise in conditions such as pregnancy, liver disease, cardiovascular problems, post-operative disorders and during some chemotherapy regimines. The geriatric patient may present with a combination of these medical problems which make drug therapy problematic.

The contraindications to the use of modified ECT are remarkably few in number. If the patient can tolerate a brief period of general anesthesia, then the only significant contraindication is the presence of raised intracranial pressure. In many texts, this contraindication is stated as the presence of a space-occupying lesion, such as a tumor, in the brain. However, the presence of a brain tumor is a relative, and not an absolute, contraindication to modified ECT.

It is instructive to list some clinical disorders which are not contraindications, despite the view of some clinicians, to the use of modified ECT. Metabolic disorders, cardiopulmonary disease, infections, other drug therapies, diseases of the muscles, bones and joints and, of course, epilepsy are not contraindications to modified ECT. If general anesthesia can be given, then, with care, ECT can be used. These points will become apparent in the later discussion of the methodology of modified ECT.

Pregnancy warrants special mentioning. The occurrence of convulsions during pregnancy, for example due to toxemia, is a reflection of the mother's primary disease. Prior to the convulsions, the fetus is suffering from this primary disorder via its hypertension and metabolic abnormalities. These primary problems are likely to have been present for a considerable time before being recognized. The fetus is also in danger secondarily from the mother's hypoxia during her tonic-clonic seizures. Convulsions which are induced by modified ECT will not have any of these problems for the mother or the fetus. Also, the fetus does not convulse and the crucial placental blood flow with its oxygen supply is not interrupted during the brief induced ECT seizure.

The third consideration for the application of modified ECT refers to the failure of other treatment modalities. Once again, it must be stressed that one is dealing with severe and critical disorders on a par with any other medical disease requiring treatment. A trial of psychotherapy or an adequate trial of psychotropic mdedications may simply not be adequately effective in removing the symptoms.

It is assumed that as part of the workup of the patient, other medical problems have to be ruled out or, if found, are being treated. Since the patient is to undergo general anesthesia they are kept "npo" in the usual manner prior to treatment. A procedure for giving modified ECT is as follows:

Atropine is administered, not specifically to reduce secretions, but rather to inhibit the parasympathetically mediated cardiac vasovagal response which occurs with a tonic-clonic convulsion of any etiology. This can be given as 1.0 milligram intravenously at the time of anesthesia. The patient is then rendered unconscious with an intravenous injection of a short-acting barbiturate such as 40 to 80 milligrams of Brevital. This should be effective in less than half a minute. A combined mouthpiece-airway can then be placed between the patient's teeth.

The unconscious patient is then given a neuromuscular blocker in order to produce a flaccid muscle paralysis throughout the body. A common choice is the depolarizing drug, Anectine, in a dose of 40 to 60 milligrams intravenously. Typically, after some 10 to 15 seconds brief fasiculations involving isolated muscle groups of the face and upper thorax will indicate the onset of action of the agent. In less than half a minute, these fasciculations will have progressed down to the feet with the result that the unconscious patient is now in a state of total flaccid paralysis.

It must be noted that this paralysis results in the patient no longer being able to breathe on his own. It is necessary that they be "bagged" during this time. However, since the rest of the procedure will take only tens of seconds, this is a simple matter.

There are a very few patients who have a relative cholinesterase deficiency which leads to a prolongation of the Anectine blockade beyond the normal duration of a few minutes. Plasma level assay of cholinesterase in order to identify such cases means a delay of days which, since urgency is a deciding factor in the use of ECT, is generally counterproductive and unacceptable. Even if the patient had this abnormality, the result would simply be that they would need respiratory assistance for an extra few minutes until the neuro-muscular blocker has been cleared from their system post-ECT.

Prior to beginning the general anesthesia, the paddles to transmit the electrical impulse should have been coated with a redux-creme to ensure good contact with the skull and the settings chosen on the ECT machine. Typically, the voltage is set between 100 to 150 volts with a pulse time of 0.5 to 1.0 seconds. This will pass a current of some 200 to 1000 milliamps into the brain which will be adequate to trigger a tonic-clonic generalized seizure. Elderly patients tend to have a somewhat higher seizure threshold and may well require higher voltages and pulse times.

The positioning of the paddles for bilateral ECT is shown schematically in the following figure.

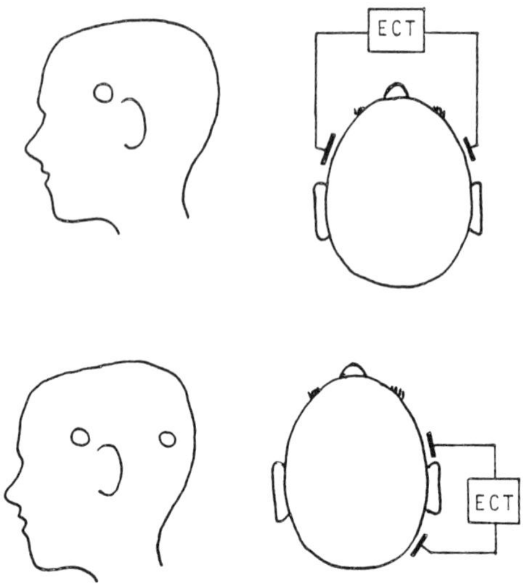

Figure 36

Therefore, as soon as the unconscious patient is in a state of flaccid paralysis, and after a couple of assisted breaths, the electrodes can be administered and the impulse delivered within a matter of seconds. The tonic phase of the generalized convulsion, because of the Anectine, involves only a slight flexion of the arms and a stiffening of the trunk for a few seconds. There is no significant body movement and certainly no "arching." The clonic phase, particularly evidenced in the lower limbs, is a mild jerking of small amplitude. The tonic-clonic features seen in idopathic generalized seizures do not occur with modified ECT because of the use of a neuromuscular agent. The "cuckoo's nest" is far from correct.

As the Anectine clears the body there may be some evidence of a Babinski reflex indicating a generalized centrencephalic convulsion. Also, as with all generalized seizures, there is some suffusion of the sclera, loss of corneal reflex, and some further dilation of the already Atropine dilated pupils.

During the tonic-clonic phase of the seizure there is a respiratory arrest. In the case of controlled ECT, this phase lasts only some 15 seconds and causes no difficulties for the patient. However, because of the remaining Anectine, the patient will not resume spontaneous respirations immediately after the clonic phase. This is simply taken care of by manual "bagging" for the next half a minute or so as the remaining Anectine is degraded.

Following the clonic phase, there will be two factors rendering the patient unconscious. Firstly, there will be the remains of the Brevital and secondly, there is the post-ictal coma associated with a generalized seizure. In general, these will be progressively reversed within a few minutes as the patient regains consciousness. Typically, this recovery follows a staggered course and is schematically shown along with the other components of the tonic-clonic convulsion in Figure 37.

There will be some patient variation in the recovery phase of modified ECT as in any case involving general anesthesia and/or a tonic-clonic convulsion. If the patient is elderly or has some organic impairment, it may take longer for the anesthetics to be eliminated and the post-ictal confusion state may be more prolonged. Examples of the post-ECT confusional state lasting more than an hour are rare. It must also be remembered that some characteristics thought to be ECT related may well be symptoms of the functional disorders for which ECT is being given.

It was stated earlier that the clinical effectiveness of the convulsive therapies depends simply on whether or not a generalized tonic-clonic seizure occurs. Also, it was noted that the clinical efficacy is not dependent on the mode of induction of the convulsion. The electrical method of induction is certainly the quickest and simplest of the available methods. Given that the voltage is adequate to propogate an impulse into the midbrain, the magnitude of the voltage is not a critical factor in the effectiveness of the therapy.

The amount of current which is propogated through the brain is a factor in the duration of the post-ECT confusion. For this reason, many clinicians prefer unilateral administration of ECT. In unilateral ECT, both electrodes are applied to the cranium containing the non-dominant hemisphere (Figure 36), which for the majority of persons is the right side of the brain.

In unilateral ECT, the electrodes should be separated by some 15 centimeters in order to ensure propogation of the electrical impulse into the critical midbrain structures rather than "shorting" between the two contact points. It is a little more difficult to ensure good electrical contact on the head of the unilateral method compared to the "pincer" effect of bilateral electrodes.

The first phase of unilateral ECT involves a partial Jacksonian seizure involving the contralateral half of the body. This becomes a secondary tonic-clonic generalized seizure when the current has propogated to involve the midbrain structures. Less current propogates in the dominant hemisphere in this technique and, as would be expected, there is less post-ECT amnesia related to the unilateral method. If done correctly, the unilateral and bilateral modified ECT procedures have equal effectiveness. The unilateral does not need more treatments than the bilateral method.

Studies sight headache as the commonest side-effect following ECT. In the course of a generalized convulsion, whether from ECT or any other cause, vasodilation of the cerebral vasculature occurs in order to increase cerebral blood flow. A result is the triggering of pain fibres located around the principle cerebral vessels and extracerebral structures such as the meningies. There are no pain fibres located in the deeper brain parencyhma as is illustrated by the fact that much stereotactic neurosurgery can be carried out with the patient conscious.

The issue of amnesia associated with ECT needs to be critically reviewed. All patients receiving a general anesthetic will have amnesia. This can be divided into three parts as is schematically shown in the following figure.

The *anterograde amnesia* includes the time the patient is fully anesthetized and the fluctuating period of recovery from the anesthetic. There is a period of amnesia which preceeds the anesthesia administration. The characteristics of this so-called *retrogade amnesia* can be illustrated by the example of a football player regaining consciousness after a collison during a game. He may report that the last thing he remembers is the kick-off and is amnesic for the flight of the ball and catching it. Later, there is, characteristically, some "shrinkage" of this retrograde amnesia and he may recall the flight of the ball and it falling into his arms but he will probably never recall the actual collison with the opposing player as he caught it.

After recovery from a general anesthetic, a patient's last memory may be of being wheeled into the operating room. Later, as the retrograde amnesia of the anesthesia is "shrunk," he may recall the anesthetist injecting the drugs into his arm. Therefore, these components of anterograde

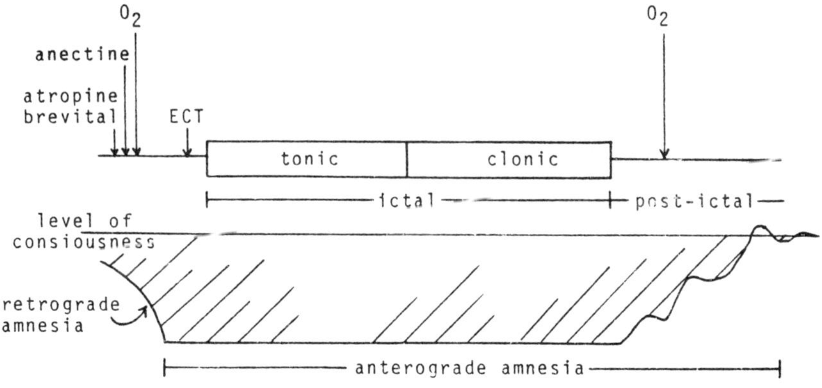

Figure 37

and retrograde amnesia are to be expected with modified ECT due to the anesthesia.

A similar amnesia profile is associated with generalized tonic-clonic seizures. This is the case no matter the etiology of this type of convulsion. Patients will remain unaware of the events during the tonic and clonic phases of the seizure, will have a patchy and fluctuating recall of events in the post-ictal recovery phase and have a short retrograde amnesic period. It is during this recovery phase component of the anterograde amnesia that the epileptic shows the confused behaviour which is often referred to as automatism.

The retrograde amnesia associated with tonic-clonic seizures has an important clinical feature if the generalized seizure is secondary to a primary focal seizure. A brain tumor, for example, may be the primary source of the epilepsy and, because of its location in the cortex, may present as a contralateral motor disorder. Since this is cortical and initially does not involve the midbrain, the patient's level of consciousness is clear. However, the seizure activity may propogate to involve centrencephalic structures causing a secondary generalized tonic-clonic convulsion with a loss of consciousness. If the propogation is rapid then these focal symptoms can be lost in the retrograde amnesia of the secondary generalized seizure. When the patient regains consciousness, he may have no recall of the focal symptoms and, if the seizure was unwitnessed, the convulsion may be thought to be a primary generalized tonic-clonic disorder. Some time later, as the retrograde amnesia of the generalized convulsion "shrinks," the patient may be able to recall the motor abnormalities and point the way to a search for the primary brain tumor.

In modified ECT, the amnesia characteristics of the anesthetic drugs and the generalized tonic-clonic seizure combine. The patient will never recall the tonic-clonic phase of the treatment. The post-ictal confusional state due to the seizure may be masked, by the sedative effects of the remaining barbiturate which, in most cases, allows the patient to "sleep through" the post-ictal phase.

Next is the question of whether or not ECT leads to irreversible amnesia by induction of brain damage. Certainly, there is an irreversible amnesia for the majority of the procedure in the same way that a patient has amnesia for an operation to remove their gallbladder and epileptics do not recall the majority of a generalised seizure. The questions really refers to whether as a direct result of ECT, patients suffer permanent "erasing of their memory banks." A number of controlled studies have been done in this regard involving the administration of standardized test-batteries to assess memory, concentration and intellectual functioning before and after ECT. These tests were given over an extended followup period. There is no objective evidence to indicate that such memory deficits occur to any significant degree.

Memory and intellectual function is frequently impaired in patients with a functional psychosis. In many cases of primary depressive disorders, these problems are prominent features of the clinical presentation. In point of fact, ECT will restore these functions to their premorbid level by treatment of the underlying disorder.

Nevertheless, there are patients who, after having ECT, attribute numerous difficulties to having had the treatments. Similarly, patients who have undergone a variety of procedures such as orthopedic surgery or chemotherapy attribute many later difficulties to these treatments. The issue is not whether such cases involving ECT, orthopedic surgery or chemotherapy can be found, but rather whether these post-treatment difficulties are a direct result of the therapy or are a psycho-social reaction to other difficulties which focuses on the treatments for a mode of rationalisation.

Most, if not all, medical treatments offer a focus for the displacement of pretreatment and subsequent concerns and difficulties. Some of these issues relate to the disease and its treatment but others are unrelated although they all become quickly amalgamated. For instance, a patient may take the position that if they had not had surgery their marriage or career would not have deteriorated. Indeed, some surgeons are reluctant to operate on certain patients because of the likelihood of them ascribing all manner of difficulties to the procedure. The patient with a "checker board" abdomen or "battleground" buttock is often viewed with caution in a preoperative consultation.

However, there are psychiatric patients whose difficulties are related to ECT and they become more debilitated after the treatments. Most of these patients have disorders such as neuroses, personality disorders, situational disturbances and adjustment reactions whilst others have organic brain syndromes. The first point is that there was little, if any, reason to have given these patients ECT since it has no proven value in the treatment of these conditions. Ironically, these patients are the ones likely predisposed to recount their ECT experience in terms of "a painful burning sensation shooting through my brain," "totally lost my personality and enjoyment of life," or "cannot remember anything any more." By acting as a displacement focus, the ECT further adds to the psycho-social problems of these patients and they are indeed worse due to having had ECT. The dramatic nature of the complaints and the person's style leads to a great deal of publicity.

Reference is sometimes made to bones being broken during ECT. The occurrence even with unmodified ECT is extremely rare. In some of these cases, the patients were elderly and had skeletal abnormalities. The tonic phase of the seizure can result in pathological torsions and stresses on some bones and the commonest reported site involved is the lower thoracic vertebrae. In modified ECT, this likelihood is eliminated since the neuromuscular blocking agents prevent these torsions and stresses by induction of a flaccid paralysis. The use of these agents makes skeletal radiographs prior to treatment generally unnecessary. Before leaving this point, one ought to ask how often patients with idiopathic generalised seizures break bones other than by falling down stairs.

The mortality associated with disorders such as primary depression has been mentioned earlier in the text. Studies of mortality during ECT combining both the unmodified and modified type, all age groups and all manner of accompanying medical complications report an occurrence of some 8 per 100,000 treatments. This is extremely small particularly in comparison to the likelihood of suicide if these disorders are not adequately treated.

The commonent cause of death during ECT is cardiac arrest. A tonic-clonic convulsion, no matter its etiology, results in the heart arresting for a few seconds in diastole. This momentary pause is due to the parasympathetically medicated vasovagal reflex. It is suggested that some of the ECT fatalities are "anesthesia" deaths due to the administration of inadequate amounts of atropine-like drugs which reduce this reflex.

Studies show that approximately half of the patients who fail to respond to a therapeutic trial of antidepressants will respond to ECT. There is still doubt as to whether this implies a subgroup of primary depression disorders which respond only to ECT and remain refractory to medications. The theoretical implications of such a situation from a neurochemical and neuropharmacological point of view are very interesting.

It is also reported that alleviation of the rank symptoms of primary depression begins earlier with ECT than with the use of antidepressants. In view of these points, and the fact that there are less medical contraindications to the use of ECT than for the antidepressants and fewer side-effects with ECT than associated with the medications, the question arises as to why ECT is not used more often in the treatment of primary depressive illness.

A major point in response to this question is that ECT offers little in terms of prophylaxis for the primary affective disorders. This is a crucial issue in the overall treatment of these disorders. The antidepressants and other psychotropic agents, such as lithium, do provide this crucial prophylactic effect.

In many clinical situations, ECT is used in the initial phase of treatment; for instance, when speed is a crucial issue in the alleviation of the symptoms. Medications such as antidepressants and lithium are introduced later when recovery is underway and prophylaxis becomes important.

An important, though unfortunate, point regarding the use of ECT is the considerable stigma associated with the procedure in the minds of some clinicians and many of the public. The repercussions of this stigma should not be underrated. The fact that the stigma is invariably based on ignorance and misunderstanding does not lessen, in fact in some instances this increases, its impact. Fortunately, in the majority of clinical cases requiring ECT, the stigma dissolves in the face of clinical needs.

On more than one occasion, ECT has been criticized because "no one knows how it works." Strickly speaking, there are few treatments in medicine whose mode of action is understood. Many treatments have elegantly proposed mechanisms whose offerings may be comforting but that is not the point. Certainly, it should not be too surprising that the neuropsychiatric disorders, with their great complexity, have proven difficult to decipher.

The relationships involving the epilepsies, in particular the limbic disorders, and the functional psychoses have been discussed earlier in the text. There is considerable experimental and clinical evidence of the inter-relations between psychotic symptomatology and cerebral dysfunction involving seizure disorders.

Earlier, in a simplified discussion, it was proposed that antidepressant drugs act by producing a relative increase in the availability of intrasynaptic neurotransmitters. There is a similar increase in biogemic amines and some amine neuro-receptors after ECT. However, this is far from being offered as an explanation of the mode of action of ECT and at this point in time, the mechanism for ECT, is not understood. However, it is hoped that it is obvious that the clinical response of certain psychotic disorders to ECT is not due to "shocking the patient into reality," "knocking them on the head to get their attention" or due to its "punative effects." It is most unfortunate that this procedure is commonly referred to as "shock treatment."

2. Tricyclic Antidepressants (TCA)

Many of the points made earlier in connection with the neuroleptics are applicable to the TCA's. In particular, the earlier outline of neurotransmitter biochemistry and the simple "single synapse" model of neuronal function can be used in a discussion of the TCA's.

The mode of action of the TCA's can be summarized as the blocking of the active re-uptake of neurotransmitters from the synaptic cleft into the presynaptic terminal. This is schematically shown in the following figure.

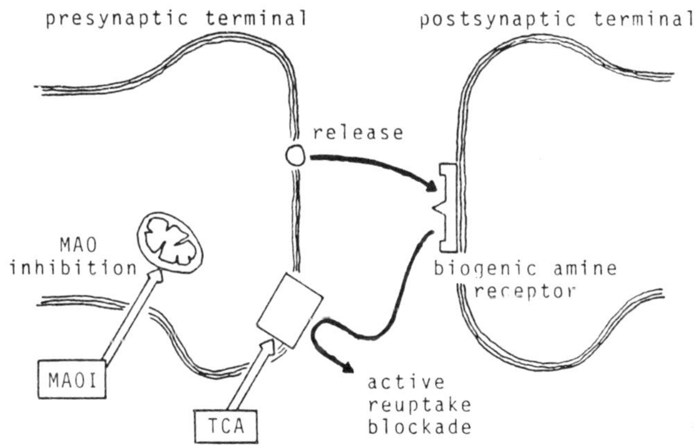

Figure 38

The result is a relative increase in synaptic neurotransmitters. Also, TCA presynaptic blockade decreases the number, but not sensitivity, of postsynaptic receptors, so-called "down regulation," particularly of beta adrenergic receptors.

As in the case of the neuroleptics, the TCA's show a variation in pharmokinetics from patient to patient which is clinically significant. Also, the TCA's have a range of side-effects which vary in occurrence and severity from patient to patient. The aim of pharmacotherapy with these drugs is to ensure an adequate therapeutic trial in each patient bearing in mind possible side-effects and the relative contraindications to their administration.

The principle route of metabolism of TCA's involves demethylation and hydroxylation by mixed function oxidases in the liver. This enzyme activity shows significant patient variability, for example, there is significant reduction of this process in many, though not all, geriatrics.

The TCA's can be divided into two groups namely, the *tertiary* and *secondary amines.* As an illustration, the tertiary TCA amitryptiline and the secondary TCA nortriptyline are schematically shown in the following figure.

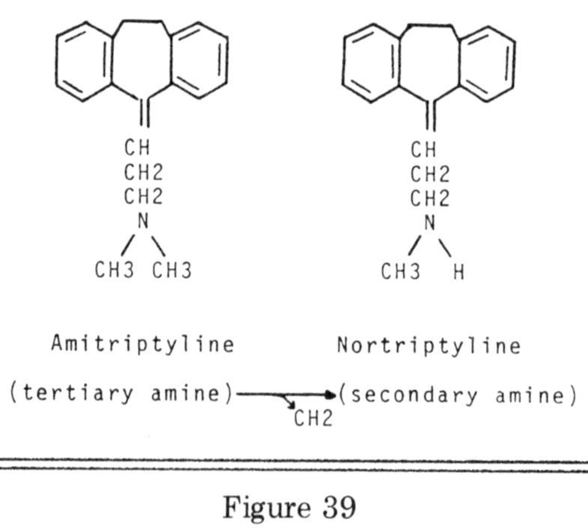

Figure 39

The similarity in structure of the TCA's with the phenothiazines should be noted. This is not too surprising since both types of medication need to "incorporate" in synaptic membranes to be clinically effective.

A percentage of ingested amitriptyline undergoes a demethylation step in the liver and is converted to nortriptyline. This conversion percentage depends on the patient's demethylation enzymes and the result is that a patient given an oral "exogenous" tertiary amine TCA will have some amount of secondary amine "endogenous" TCA in their blood stream.

This does not mean that patients prescribed tertiary amine TCA "get two tricyclic antidepressants for the price of one." For some patients, this demethylation percentage is minimal but for others it may be such that essentially all of the parent TCA is converted into a secondary amine derivative. There is no methylation step which converts secondary amine TCA's into tertiary medications. Patients who are prescribed nortriptyline do not produce "endogenous" amitriptyline.

The plasma half-life of TCA's varies noticably from patient to patient but typically, the half-life is from 24 to 36 hours. There are a number of diseases, for instance liver disorders, which can significantly alter the TCA half life. This alteration is usually in the direction of an increase in the plasma-half life indicating TCA "hypometabolism." Geriatric patients warrant special attention since they have, in general, some impairment of the liver enzymes which breakdown TCA and are more likely to have other accompanying medical disorders which can slowdown the TCA pharmacokinetics.

The liver is the principle site of metabolism for many medications and the enzymes involves in the breakdown of the TCA's are required in the handling of these other drugs. Barbiturates, alcohol, chloral hydrate and oral contraceptives are some medications which will lower the plasma concentration of TCA's. Neuroleptics and analeptics, such as amphetamine, will raise the plasma concentration of TCA's. It appears that some of the benzodiazepines have little influence on the plasma concentration and half-life of TCA's by virtue of their minimal effects on the liver's microenzymal system.

Assuming that the diagnosis of a major depressive disorder warranting treatment with a TCA has been made, then an issue is the choice of TCA which from a clinical point of view involves a number of considerations. Firstly, if the patient's presenting symptom profile features a particular symptom or two, is one TCA more indicated than another?

For instance, it has been said that amitriptyline is specifically indicated when a dominant symptom is insomnia. Imipramine has been sighted as the TCA of choice when there is notable lassitude and anergia in the depressive profile. For those patients who display prominent obsessive-compulsive features, chlorimipramine has been suggested as the preferred TCA.

The more commonly used TCA's are schematically shown in the following figure. There is a striking similarity in their structures to one another and to the phenothiazines. It is not surprising that they have many side-effects in common with the neuroleptics.

However, it is surprising that by making a small alteration in TCA's structure one can "focus" on a particular symptom of the depressive profile. It may well be that the suggestion of a particular TCA for a given symptom is a result of the symptoms of the patients included in the particular studies that lead to these conclusions or the method of analysis of the data.

Perhaps choosing between the TCA's is better based on their relative side-effects than on symptom specificity. Therefore, a second question is whether or not there is a significant difference in the side-effects of the different tricyclic antidepressants? At this point, it becomes necessary to outline the common side-effects of the TCA's.

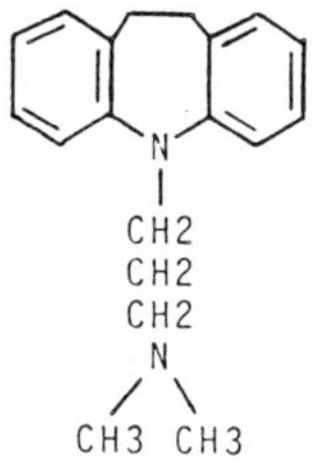

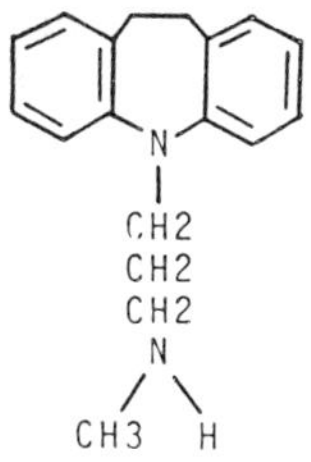

Imipramine Desipramine

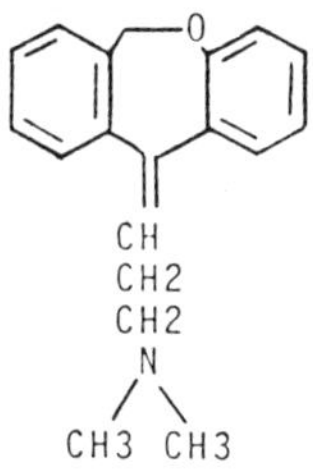

Doxepin

Figure 40

1. Dystonia

Acute dystonic reactions such as torticollis, opisthotonos and occular gyric crisis are very uncommon due to TCA's. Isolated cases have been reported but these side-effects are not a feature of the TCA's.

2. Parkinsonian-Like Syndromes and Extrapyramidal Symptoms

The TCA's do not have the post-synaptic dopamine receptor blocking action that is associated with the neuroleptics. However, it should be recognized that symptoms akin to akinesia and petit march as well as a "mask-like" facies can occur during TCA treatment.

These symptoms in association with TCA's are likely to be a more generalised drug induced effect than blockade at the corpus striatum. They could be a reflection of sedation or could, in fact, be symptoms of the major depressive disorder which are being unmasked by the drug therapy.

In addition to entering the central nervous system, the TCA's effect peripheral nerves and can result in mono and poly neuropathies. Paresthesia and lower motor neuron palsies can be induced as well as tremors of both the at-rest and action type.

Dyskinesias similar to akasthesia can occur during treatment with TCA's, however, these symptoms are likely to be an expression of the patient's depression, anxiety and agitation. Nevertheless, their occurrence should lead to the consideration of a possible TCA neurotoxicity. There is no indication for the use of anticholinergics in the treatment of any of these disorders if they are TCA induced. It is best to consider an alteration in the prescribed dosage or changing to another TCA in the hope that the side-effects are an idiosyncratic reaction to the particular TCA.

3. Anticholinergic Effects

TCA's have a range of significant anticholinergic side-effects. Many of these are identical to those outlined earlier in association with the neuroleptics and so, at this point only some of them will be discussed.

It is almost invariable that patients receiving TCA's will experience a dry mouth early in the course of treatment. In most cases, this effect diminishes after a week or so but in some patients it persists throughout treatment.

Another frequent and early complaint during TCA treatment is a blurring of vision due to loss of accommodation. As in the case of it's occurence with neuroleptic therapy, there is no specific treatment but in many cases there is some compensation and adjustment during the course by the autonomic system. Sustained dilation of the pupils due to anticholinergic side-effects could impair intraoccular drainage and be a problem for patients with glaucoma. However, unless the pre-existing glaucoma was severe or of acute onset, raised intraoccular pressure is not a significant contraindication to the use of TCA's.

Constipation is a common side-effect of TCA's but it must be remembered that bowel symptoms, such as gas cramps and reduced bowel movements are often symptoms of the depressive profile. Complaints and concerns involving the bowel are a common feature of hypochondriasis in major depressive illness. It is possible that this symptom will decrease as the TCA's become effective in ameliorating the depressive illness. It would be unfortunate if the treatment were discontinued unnecessarily, and for this reason, it is well to make an assessment of the so-called drug related side-effects before the patient is begun on TCA treatment.

Difficulties with micturation can often arise but acute urinary retention is rare. Prostatic hypertrophy is not a contraindication to the use of TCA's if the clinical presentation warrants. Impotency is a relatively common symptom associated with the depressive syndrome as an expression of a loss in sexual drive. The patient may displace his inability to sustain an erection onto a TCA side-effect, for example hypotension, but this is unlikely to be the case in the absence of other neurovascular side-effects.

Accumulation of anticholinergic side-effects, as in the case of the neuroleptics, can result in a drug-induced cholinergic psychosis. This is more likely to be seen in the elderly. Specifically, the levels of acetycholine, an important neurotransmitter, tend to be significantly low in geriatrics. This appears to be due to a relative deficiency in choline acetyltransferase which is necessary in the conversion of choline to acetylcholine. Therefore, drugs with significant anticholinergic properties such as TCA's and neuroleptics tend to be poorly tolerated by many of these patients.

4. Cardiovascular Effects

Orthostatic hypotension is frequently induced by TCA's, the most likely mechanism being alpha-adrenergic blockade. It is often prudent to warn patients of possible transient dizziness and syncopal episodes.

For some patients, this fall in blood pressure is troublesome and it is not compensated for as treatment continues. It may be necessary to divide the required daily dosage into a number of administration spaced throughout the day. For others, the taking of the daily dose at bedtime means that the transient hypotensive effects occur when they are in bed and, perhaps, asleep. For most patients, these orthostatic hypotensive episodes diminish after a few weeks on the medication.

Probably the most important side-effects of the TCA's involve the heart. These side-effects pose, perhaps, the major problems associated with the prescribing of TCA for the treatment of major depressive disorders. The relative cardiac effects of the various TCA's are often a major consideration in the choosing of one TCA in preference to the others for the treatment of the patient.

All TCA's at dosages required for antidepressant effects influence, to some degree, the contractility of the myocardium. In patients with recent and extensive myocardial damage, the use of TCA's is precluded for a number of weeks, or perhaps much longer, until the cardiovascular system has stabilised. Under this circumstance, the patient's acute depressive syndrome can be safely treated with ECT. There may still be a problem of prophylaxis at a later date which will likely require the use of TCA's.

The TCA's have a significant quinidine-like effect on the cardiac conduction system. This impairment of intracardiac conduction is the main cardiotoxic effect of the TCA's. This blockade can be illustrated by considering the progressive blockade due to a TCA overdose which, if treated, can be fatal.

It is said that as many as 40 percent of overdose patients who need to spend some time in an intensive care unit have taken an overdose of TCA's. This is a depressing statistic. One wonders how many of these patients were inappropriately prescribed TCA's simply because they had the symptom of depression? That is to say, how many were given the drug when, in fact, it would not have any meaningful benefit?

Typically, an overdose of 1.5 to 2.0 grams of TCA's such as amitriptyline, imipramine and the others, will be a major threat to life. It should be noted that obtaining such a potentially lethal quantity is not difficult. For, example, a prescription for 50 mg of amitriptyline as a hypnotic will have sufficient for a suicide with one month's supply. It is unfortunate that the TCA is used for treatment of a symptom probably unrelated to a major depressive illness but provides a suicidal vehicle. That is to say, the wrong drug for the wrong disorder for the wrong reason in the wrong dose.

Within an hour or so of swallowing a couple of grams of TCA, the person becomes obtunded, slurred and ataxic. Shortly after this, generalized convulsions can occur and the patient may move into a non-responsive drug induced coma. From the time of ingestion, progressive changes take place involving the patient's cardiac status. The initial response is likely to be a tachycardia to compensate for the orthostatic hypotension. As the quinidine effect of the TCA increases, it will be reflected as a prolongation of the PR, QRS, and QT segments on the electrocardiogram.

The QT interval is of particular value in demonstrating the conduction blockade. It should be noted that prolongation of the QT interval can be masked on the EKG if there is a tachycardia. This is often the case in the early stages of TCA overdose. In these circumstances, it is necessary to calculate a corrected QT interval (QTc) in order to identify the prolonged conduction time.

Additional evidence of cardiac compromise at this time includes non-specific ST changes such as suppression and inversion indicating myocardial ischemia and strain. The next step in this progressive blockade focuses on changes in the distal bundle of His. There are runs of aberrant beats, for example PVC's, and arrythmias including ventricular tachycardia.

In therapeutic doses, the TCA's quinidine-like effects may control isolated PVC's which the patient may have from a pre-existing cardiac disorder. The existence of limited runs of PVC's is not a contraindication to beginning treatment with TCA's if the patient has a major depressive illness although one would not suggest that TCA's be used specifically for this purpose. The occurrence of such abberrant beats in overdose cases is, of course, a different matter.

The final and crucial step in the progressive blockage of a TCA overdose is the onset of bradycardia and, finally, asystole. The change from a ventricular tachycardia to bradycardia and finally asystole implies that the blockade of this distal bundle of His has progressed to completeness.

The progression from simple tachycardia through ventricular arrythmia to bradycardia and arrest can take less than an hour depending on the severity of the overdose and

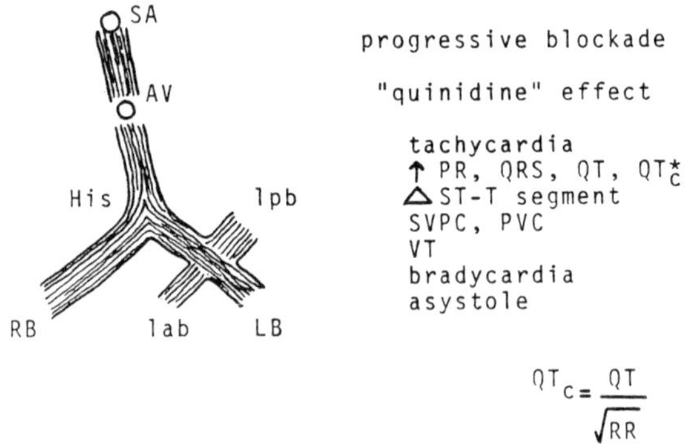

Figure 41

the patient's pre-existing cardiovascular status. There is a likelihood that because of the progressive nature of the cardiac difficulties they may go unrecognised in the early stages. To begin with, the patient may be a "well-known psych case" who is often "OD-ing for attention." If he arrives, for the third time that month, slightly obtunded and tachycardic then, in a busy emergency room, he may well be left somewhat unattended after the initial examination. Within a short time, the progressive conduction blockade can move from artial tachycardia to cardiac arrest.

The blockade of the distal bundle of His by TCA's is of a depolarizing type which makes the heart essentially non-responsive to any compensatory changes attempted by the autonomic nervous system. This means that the TCA induced bradycardia, should the progressive toxicity go this far, cannot be adequately reversed by giving other medications. It is necessary to have installed a mechanical pacer for these problems. Therefore, once ventricular arrythmias appear and upcoming bradycardia is sensed, then installation of such a device may be a wise move in the clinical management.

Since most of the TCA side-effects are anticholinergic, the anticholinesterase drugs have been suggesed to attenuate these problems. It should be noted that some anticholinesterases do not effectively cross the blood brain barrier and will have little, if any, use in the alleviation of many of the troublesome TCA side-effects.

The anticholinesterase physostigmine salicylate crosses the blood brain barrier and a couple of milligrams given intravenously will quickly reverse TCA side-effects such as blurred vision, dry mouth and drowsiness. However, the drug has a half-life in the central nervous system of some 10 minutes so that it is impractical in terms of alleviating these side-effects for prolonged periods. Furthermore, many of these side-effects will diminish during treatment with the TCA's and if they do not, they are small inconveniences when compared to the rank symptoms of the primary depression.

The use of anticholinesterases in the management of a TCA overdose is of interest. It may well be that a single intravenous administration of physostigmine will reverse any obnumbulation and slurred speech for some minutes and allow clarification of the history which may prove to be valuable in the overall management of the patient. However, there are problems inherent in repeated administration of an anticholinesterase if the overdose is of sufficient magnitude that blockade of the distal bundle of His resulting in bradycardia and arrest eventually occurs. The accumulation of anticholinergic effects may, by potentiation of the vagal tone, increase the likelihood of cardiac arrest. The initial use of this drug to clarify the history may prove to be "expensive" at a later time in the management if indeed the patient took a life threatening overdose.

The best management of TCA overdose begins with taking the situation seriously and recognizing that the cardiotoxic effects of these drugs follows a progressive course. Obviously, gastric lavage needs to be performed and the patient's cardiopulmonary status carefully monitored. If the progressive quinidine effects on the cardiac conduction system are seen, then decisions must be made in terms of the need for a demand type pacemaker.

In most cases, given the typical half-life of these medications, the patients will be out of critical danger within 24 to 36 hours. Even then there is likely to be indications of some cardiotoxicity remaining by virtue of the prolonged QTc interval.

The major question in terms of TCA therapy is whether some TCA's are significantly less cardiotoxic than others. Certainly, a TCA with little cardiotoxicity at dosages required to produce a therapeutic response would be preferred. Also, given the frequent risk of suicide in many of these patients, a TCA with low cardiotoxic potential would be valuable.

Furthermore, one is frequently faced with a patient who, in addition to a primary depressive illness, has significant pre-existing cardiovascular disease. In particular, this is seen in geriatrics since they are more likely to have cardiovascular disease than younger people. If the cardiac problems are stabler and not acute, then even marked problems such as extensive ishemia and infarction, as well as bundle branch blocks and simple arrythmias, are not a contraindication to the judicious use of TCA's in treating their primary depressive illness. A major concern is that given the increased likelihood of idiosyncratic pharmokinetics in geriatrics one has to be sure that they are not given unnecessarily high or homeopathic doses of the TCA's.

There have been a number of studies investigating the effects of various TCA's on patients with non-acute cardiac disease. The early reports focused on the relatively low cardiac problems of doxepin hydrochloride. However, when the studies are reviewed critically, this TCA is not significantly less cardiotoxic than the others. All the TCA's can be given in amounts required to produce a therapeutic response without producing untoward cardiotoxicity in the majority of patients. There are certainly some patients who show an extreme response involving orthostatic hypotension, alterations in the cardiac conduction, a dry mouth or blurred vision, however, given the complexity of the TCA pharmokinetics and the many factors which influence the handling of the TCA's by the body's organ system such idiosyncracies are to be expected.

Therefore, it appears that the TCA's form a relatively uniform group of drugs in terms of clinical response and side-effects with the differences being more a reflection of idiosyncracies than specific properties making one TCA "better than the others." The classicial profile regarding side-effects for the TCA's is given in the following Table. It is questionable that a definitive choice between the various drugs can be made on the basis of the table's overgeneralised information.

Despite the idiosyncracies of pharmokinetics, to say nothing of the nature of the clinical manifestation of primary depressive illness, one can propose "typical" dosages for the TCA's required to produce a therapeutic response.

	mg per day	hypo-BP	antichol
Tertiary TCA			
imipramine (Tofranil)	200-300	high	intermed
amitriptyline (Elavil)	200-300	high	high
doxepin HCl (Sinequan)	200-300	intermed	intermed
Secondary TCA			
nortriptyline (Pamelor)	100-150	intermed	intermed
desipramine (Norpramin)	200-300	intermed	intermed
"second generation"			
maprotiline (Ludiomil)	200	intermed	low
trazodone (Desyrel)	300	low	none?
amoxapine (Asendin)	300	intermed	intermed
nomifensine (Merital)	150	low	low

Table 5

This data is based on controlled clinical trials. Compilation of data from these studies allows that if a primary depressive disorder is given an adequate therapeutic trial of TCA's, then there is some 70 percent chance of alleviating the clinical symptoms. This figure indicates the effectiveness of these medications when they are properly used in the treatment of the correct disorder. It is instructive to compare this figure with pharmacotherapy of other medical disorders. A frequent occurrence after such a comparison is a rethinking of notions concerning psychiatric treatments.

If one calculates the P value for these controlled studies of TCA's in the treatment of primary depressive disorders, it is a miniscule number of the order of 10^{-25}. This means the success of the TCA's can be accounted for by "chance" as a fraction with some 25 zeros in its denominator. In fact the P value is akin to that of studies involving antibiotics and their treatment of bacteria infections. It is tragic that such a "powerful" class of drugs is so frequently misused, and perhaps indicates that psychopharmacology has outstripped many clinicians' notions of the subject. The "typical" daily dose of the common TCAs to provide an adequate therapeutic trial are given in the preceeding table.

As an illustration of establishing and carrying through an adequate therapeutic trial, we will consider the secondary amine TCA nortriptyline. From the previous table, the indication is that the typical required daily dose is from 100 to 150 milligrams orally. Since the half-life is some 24 to 36 hours, then the total dose can be given in a single administration, for example at bedtime, and will achieve steady state conditions after approximately one week on this daily dosage.

The aim, as in the case of the neuroleptics in the alleviation of schizophrenic symptoms, is to titrate the medication against the clinical symptomatology of the primary depressive disorder. In schizophrenia, this is a relatively easy task with the acute disorder because of the florrid and relatively non-entrenched symptomatology. It is a much more difficult undertaking in subacute or chronic schizophrenia because the symptoms are somewhat masked and more entrenched so that symptom recovery is a slower and less obvious process. The nature of the symptomatology of primary depressive illness makes TCA titration more akin with the neuroleptic titration in chronic rather than acute schizophrenias.

A depressed patient may show significant signs of improvement soon after hospitalisation and before commencement of TCA's. This reflects the important psychological and sociological factors of the depressive illness and their contribution to the overall therapy. The fact that a patient shows an immediate improvement of the rank symptoms of the depressive syndrome with the commencement of TCAs does not mean that the TCAs are responsible. These changes are likely to be a placebo response and in many instances it is worthwhile pointing this out to the patient since this early improvement is unlikely to be sustained or continued.

Typically, the nortriptyline will begin its "real" effect within three or four days. Often, the first symptom to revert is the sleep disturbance. It is interesting that the patient may not sleep longer with the TCA but they describe a more "beneficial and restful night's sleep." One should allow at least a week to ten days before considering a change in the dose of the nortriptyline. It has taken six or seven days to reach a steady state plasma level and there has been an equivalent delay in "getting into the presynaptic terminal membrane to block active reuptake of neurotransmitter at the critical cerebral sites."

If at this point the symptom profile is beginning to be resolved and the patient is showing steady signs of overall clinical improvement, then there is no indication to alter the TCA dosage. In general terms, the nortriptyline should be run for two to three weeks to maximise its clinical effectiveness. If there is an "arrest" in the improvement, or if a set of symptoms prove to be refractory to treatment, one may consider an increase in the dosage to 125 or 150 milligrams. This change in dosage begins a "second step" in titration of a week to ten days duration.

In summary, one is titrating the dosage from the 100 milligram starting point in steps of a week to ten days duration. This step interval allows time for the medication to have an effect on the symptom profile and time for these changes to be identified in the clinical interview.

The pharmacotherapy can be summarised as an adequate dose of a TCA for sufficient time establishing a therapeutic trial to alleviate the clinical symptoms bearing in mind the TCA's possible side-effects and relative contraindications. This may sound rather "wordy" but it is better than "a couple of days on a TCA at a dose chosen from the PDR to see if the patient can get happy again." The recommended form of this type of therapeutic trial, even with a two dosage adjustment has a span of some three weeks. This does not constitute an unnecessarily prolonged hospitalisation for the treatment of a major depressive episode.

It is likely that some geriatric patients will metabolise TCA's at a reduced rate compared with younger patients. However, as in the case of neuroleptic medications, this point should not be applied as an absolute rule in designing a therapeutic trial for elderly patients.

Patients, both young and elderly, may have accompanying problems such as hepatic or cardiovascular disease which can significantly alter TCA pharmokinetics. Also, a given patient may be receiving any one of a range of drugs which can markedly alter TCA metabolism. These idiosyncracies in pharmokinetics may result in hypometabolism or hypermetabolism of the TCA's. This can lead to either significantly longer or shorter plasma half lifes for the TCA with possible toxic or homeopathic amounts of medication respectively.

Therefore, in patients where one of these abnormal metabolism situations may exist the titration of the TCA, for example nortriptyline, could be initiated with a dosage of 50 or 75 milligrams per day rather than 100 or 150 milligrams. The previously described "steps" can be followed and it is likely that duration of the necessary trial need not be significantly prolonged.

If after an adequate therapeutic trial of TCA the patient does not respond sufficiently well, then it becomes necessary to reaccess the case. Assuming that the diagnosis of a primary depressive illness still holds, then a change of TCA is indicated. Some two or three days after discontinuing the first TCA the second choice can be safely administered.

It may well be that the partial failure of the first TCA trial now introduces a factor of urgency into the case. This may call for the use of ECT rather than beginning a second TCA.

At the time of discharge from hospital, the patient should remain on the TCA dosage which maximised the clinical response in the hospital. In many respects, discharge is stressful for the patient, for instance, they return to psychosocial problems some of which were likely to have been factors in the original problem. Therefore, at discharge, it is unwise to introduce the variable of an alteration in the patient's medication.

The outpatient treatment immediately following discharge is crucial in terms of the illness's overall prognosis. Certainly, the patient should be seen a number of times during the first couple of weeks in order to assess their symptom profile and the psychosocial circumstances.

If after a month or so the patient has continued to function well and is reintegrating into the family and work environment without any reemergence of the depressive syndrome, then one could consider a reduction in dosage of the TCA. The patient's past psychiatric history is of great importance in making this decision, for instance, if the patient has had more than one depressive episode then the question of the need for a prolonged pharmacological prophylaxis arises.

In the case of recurrent unipolar episodes, continuing the TCA for longer than a few months before beginning a gradual reducing titration is advisable. It may well be that the patient cannot be totally taken off the TCA without a reemergence of some depressive symptomatology and so must remain on the medication for an extended time.

In the case of recurrent bipolar disorders, it may be necessary to continue to treat the patient prophylactically with lithium carbonate. This point will be discussed in more detail later in this chapter when lithium therapy is reviewed. It should also be mentioned that lithium may be a useful prophylactic agent for the recurring unipolar disorder and in some cases preferable to continued maintainence with TCAs.

Care should be taken in the followup of a previously depressed patient receiving a TCA to identify any subsequent manic symptoms. One would be specifically aware of this possibility in a patient who had a previous manic episode, however, it should be recalled that many bipolar patients do not present a manic episode until their second or third relapse. The type of prophylaxis and how long it should be continued remains in a large part a matter of informed clinical judgment.

As in any branch of medicine, numerous attempts have been made to find "litmus" tests to help diagnose psychiatric disorders and aid in the prescribing and administration of medication. Some of these tests will be discussed in the following section.

a. Dexamethasone Suppression Test (DST)

Cortisol secretion has a circadian rhythm. The normal pattern shows a steady decrease after 4:00 pm to the lowest level of the cycle at midnight. After 12:00 pm, the secreation of cortisol begins to rise and reaches its maximum level around 9:00 am.

The control of cortisol secretion involves the hypothalamic-pituitary-adrenal (HPA) axis. The HPA axis is under the influence of numerous complex feedback loops one of which involves the corticotropin releasing factor, adrenocorticotropic hormone (ACTH) and cortisol level.

The HPA axis interfaces with the limbic system therefore if the major affective disorders relate to disturbances of the limbic system they will disturb the HPA axis. In particular, a disturbance of the limbic system may be reflected as a distortion of the cortisol circadian rhythm.

The biochemical theories of depression propose a relative deficiency of the principle neurotransmitters, namely, norepinephrine, serotonin and dopamine. These neurotransmitters influence the HPA axis at a number of points, one of these involves cortisol. Therefore, one has a possible link between the biochemical theories of depression and a hormone which can be manipulated and measured. This, in a sense, offers means of "tapping" into the functional limbic system. For instance, norepinephrine has an inhibiting effect on the HPA axis and its circadian rhythm is a mirror image of that of cortisol. Serotonin has an activating effect on the HPA axis and its circadian rhythm follows that of cortisol. The norepinephrine deficent depressions may have a "high" cortisol whilst the serotonin deficent depressions may be due to suppression by a "high" cortisol.

Administration of a synthetic glucocorticoid will suppress the hypothalamic production of corticotropin releasing factor causing a decreased production of ACTH in the pituitary which in turn results in a decrease in the adrenal output of cortisol. This represents the normal inhibitory HPA axis feedback for the control of cortisol.

The oral administration of 1.0 milligram of dexamethasone at 11:00 pm or midnight will result in the suppression of cortisol secretion over the next twenty four hours. Specifically, the plateau of cortisol secretion between 4:00 pm and midnight the day following the dexamethasone administration should have cortisol levels below 5 microgram/dl as measured by radioimmunossay or 4 microgram/dl determined by competative protein binding. This normal dexamethasone suppression is schematically shown in the following figure.

It was found that patients with primary depressive disorders had a large percentage of abnormal cortisol suppressions following this oral administration of dexamethasone. These patients failed to suppress to the degree seen in normal controls. These so-called *positive* DST patients had a responsive HPA axis but it was less sensitive to dexamethasone suppression.

The DST is schematically shown in the previous figure. The protocol involves giving 1.0 milligram of oral dexamethasone at 11:00 pm and measuring the plasma cortisol at 8:00 am, 4:00 pm and 11:00 pm the following day. A positive DST has these plasma cortisols greater than 5 microgram/dl by radioimmune assay or 4 microgram/dl by compatative protein binding assay.

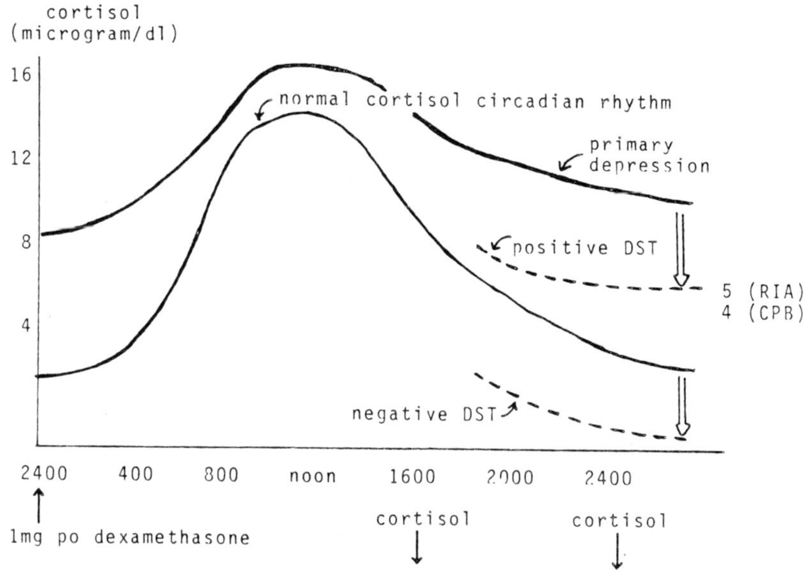

Figure 42

Clearly, there are a number of problems. Firstly, not without a degree of cynicism, this is a remarkably "simple" test for such a "complex" problem as the neuroendrocrine-neuropsychiatric disorders. One has to be somewhat skeptical about "deciding on the overall architecture of a building by looking at one brick" but on the other hand it may be "elegant" rather than "simple." Secondly, the cortisol assays are not without problems and one is concerned with small incremental changes in deciding whether or not there has been a failure to suppress and hence a positive DST. However, the main concern is whether these cortisol changes are a "marker" of the major depressive disorder or rather they reflect secondary changes. If it is the latter, then the cortisol profile is a reflection of the "turmoil" rather than a "marker" of the specific disorder of a primary depressive disorder.

The hope would be that the positive DST would have a marked *sensitivity* for primary depressive disorders and in addition it would have *specificity* for these disorders. That is to say a high percentage of patients with the clinical diagnosis of a primary depressive illness would show a positive DST by their failure of suppression but a positive DST would be rare in other psychiatric disorders, for instance, schizophrenia and the atypical, reactive and secondary depressive disorders.

The results of controlled studies of the DST are encouraging. The primary depressive disorders show a positive DST, that is failure of suppression, in some 50 to 85 per cent of the patients. In addition, the occurrence of a positive DST in patients with disorders other than primary depression is very low ranging from 0 to 15 percent. It would appear that from the early studies the DST has both a sensitivity and specificity.

At this point, it can be said that the DST has clinical value in distinguishing the primary depressive disorder from secondary depressive disorders due to, for example, schizophrenia, neuroses, adjustment reactions and substance abuse. It does not appear that the DST can distinguish between the primary depressive disorders of the unipolar and bipolar type.

However, there is still a large percentage of patients with a primary depressive disorder, as many as 50 percent, who will suppress and show a negative DST. Therefore, it must be stressed that the DST is not a "litmus" test for the diagnosis of primary depressive disorders. It is an adjunct to the clinical diagnosis procedure and it must not be used in place of this examination. After all, one does not diagnose rheumatoid arthritis on the single point of the RF preparation and it is "simple" in comparison to the neuropsychiatric disorders of depression.

The DST may have a value in plotting the progress of pharmacotherapy. If the patient has a positive DST and because of the additional clinical information a TCA is given, the course of the recovery may be followed by repeating the DST. It may be that the DST converts to one of suppression earlier in the course of treatment than the symptoms show significant change by clinical interview. It may be that conversion of the DST offers an early indication that the medications are being effective. On the other hand, a persistantly positive DST along with only a partial recovery of the clinical symptoms may suggest that the clinician change to another TCA in the hope of a more complete response.

b. TCA Reuptake Blockade

The TCA's differ in their relative ability to block the reuptake of various neurotransmitters at the presynaptic membrane. If the primary depressive disorders can be differentiated in terms of being a serotonin or norepinephrine deficiency, then one type of TCA may be preferrable to another. The relative blockade of the amine pump for some of the common TCAs is given in the following table.

	Amine Pump Blockade			
	NE		5HT	D
Prototype				
imipramine	mod		mod	-
amitriptyline	mod	<	mod	-
nortriptylinc	mod	>	mod	-
desipramine	mod	>	mod	-
Second generation				
trazodone	-		mod	-
nomifensine	-		-	mod

Table 6

Amphetamine challenges have been suggested to differentiate the norepinephrine from the serotonin deficient depressions. In simple terms, patients who showed a clinical response to a couple of days on a low oral dose of amphetamine were found to have low pretreatment urinary MHPG levels. The low urinary MHPG levels was taken to signify that they have a norepinephrine deficent depression and so would have a better response to a TCA which showed a preference for blockade of the norepinephrine amine pump. These patients were found to respond very well to desipramine and not to amitriptyline. Patients who did not respond to a short trial of amphetamine were found to have a normal or elevated pretreatment urinary MHPG level. These depressive disorders responded better to amitriptyline than desipramine.

The implication of these data is that a short amphetamine challenge may indicate the choice of the TCA for the main therapeutic trial. The serotonin versus norepinephrine split of the primary depressive disorders is an oversimplification and it should not be expected that such as the amphetamine challenge would be more than a contributing point in choosing a TCA for a given case.

c. TCA Plasma Level Determinations

A key factor in using TCA's in the treatment of primary depression is ensuring an adequate therapeutic trial. The trial should be of a sufficient duration and employ an optimal dose of medication.

It may very well be that ensuring an adequate therapeutic trial is more important in terms of the outcome of treatment than in choosing a particular TCA on the basis of associated side-effects, selective amine pump blockade or neurotransmitter urinary metabolite determinations.

The idiosyncracies of TCA pharmokinetics from patient to patient and the individualisation of associated side-effects was discussed in detail earlier in this chapter. The "step-wise" titration of a TCA during a therapeutic trial was also discussed and it was proposed that such a protocol allowed some tailoring of drug to the given patient. Nevertheless, even employing a titration technique, there is a likelihood of not identifying patients with marked idiosyncracies in pharmokinetics for up to weeks into treatment. The use of plasma level determinations allows for a quicker identification of the hypo or hypermetaboliser of a TCA.

Factors such as age, medications being prescribed for other conditions and additional medical problems such as liver disease can significantly influence TCA pharmokinetics. Therefore, the use of plasma levels can add an important safety factor to the use of TCAs since the resultant influence of these factors can be determined for a given patient.

Although plasma levels can increase the safety and make for a more exact tailoring of dosage for a given patient, it must not be taken to mean that these levels provide a "litmus" test for adequate therapy. It does not follow that because a patient is "in the therapeutic range" then their clinical response to that TCA has been maximised. Plasma levels provide a useful guide to therapy but, as in the case of the DST, they do not provide a "short cut."

The first point raised in connection with plasma levels is whether or not the values correlate to the clinical findings in term of clinical response? Reports have been published on the relationship of plasma levels to clinical response for several of the commonly prescribed TCAs and a summary of this information is given in the following table.

A number of studies do not find a correlation between clinical response and plasma concentration and for some TCA's there have been insufficient studies to draw a conclusion. However, in the case of some TCA's there is sufficient data to allow the demarcation of so-called *therapeutic range* and *limits.* However, even if no therapeutic ranges can be defined the plasma levels can still be of significant use in identifying patients with significantly abnormal TCA pharmokinetics.

Tertiary amine	Therapeutic Range (ng/ml)
amitriptyline + nortriptyline	75-200
imipramine + desipramine	150-300
doxepin + D-methyldox	90-250
Secondary amine	
nortriptyline	50-150
desipramine	20-160

Table 7

Tertiary amine TCAs undergo demethylation to secondary amines at a rate which varies with the individual (Figure 39). Amitriptyline and imipramine are demethylated to nortriptyline and desmipramine respectively and each of these secondary amine metabolities are clinically effective TCAs in their own right. Patients treated with tertiary TCAs hence have an individualised ratio of two TCAs in their blood stream depending on their demethylation enzyme activity. There is an "exogenous"tertiary amine parent and an "endogenous" secondary amine offspring. The determination of the clinically effective plasma level concentration for tertiary TCAs is somewhat problematic. Certainly, one does not get "two for the price of one" and the resultant level is not simply the addition of the "parent and offspring" plasma levels.

Administration of secondary amine TCA's as the parent compound does not present this problem since they do not undergo a methylation step to an endogenous tertiary amine TCA. Therefore, the laboratory report will be of a single value and interpretation is simpler. The secondary amines do have other metabolities which can have a clinical effect, for example, the 10-hydroxy metabolite of nortriptyline. However, since these levels are not reported by standard laboratories and their clinical effects are small these compounds will be neglected in this discussion.

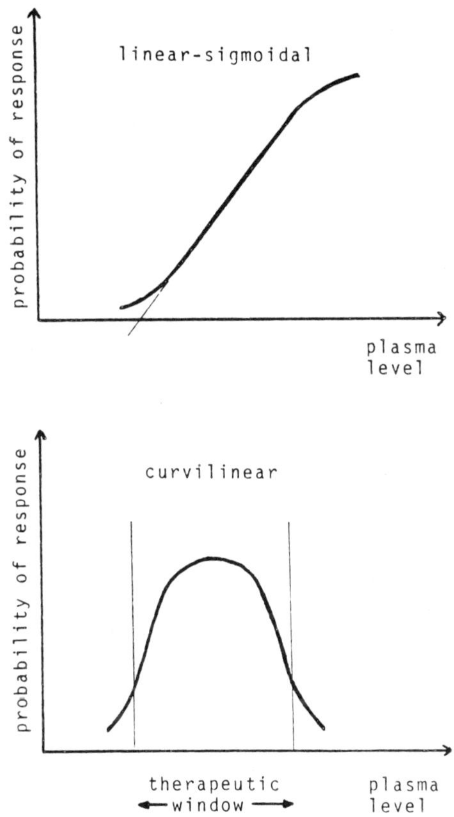

Figure 43

Curves showing the relationship of TCA plasma level to clinical response for adequately investigated TCA's are of two types. One is the *curvilinear* as shown in the preceeding figure. The probability of a clinical response to the TCA follows as inverted U with the plasma concentration as the abscissa.

The probability of a clinical response is low for plasma level concentrations less than a cut-off value, which in the case of nortriptyline is some 50 ng/ml. This does not mean that a patient will not respond to nortriptyline on an oral dose which results in a plasma level of, for example, 35 ng/ml but that the probability of such an occurrence is very low. The probability of response increases along with the rising plasma level concentration and then it peaks and falls. This allows for the definition of an upper cut-off plasma concentration above which the probability of clinical response is once again very low. In the case of nortriptyline, this upper limit is around 150 ng/ml. These upper and lower plasma levels allow for the demarcation of a *therapeutic window* for TCAs with a curvilinear relationship of response probability and plasma level.

The second type of relationship is the *linear or sigmoidal* curve as shown in Figure 43. Again, a minimal plasma level is necessary before clinical improvement can be expected, and the probability of a response increases as the plasma concentration rises. The probability of response then plateaus but an upper limit is not defined as in the case of the curvilinear relationship.

It should be noted that the downturn of response probability in the curvilinear group, with subsequent defining of an upper level of the therapeutic window, and the plateauing of the sigmoidal group are not reflections of TCA toxicity or the onset of drug induced side-effects. These features are inherent characteristics of the pharmokinetics and efficacy of the various TCAs.

The linear or sigmoidal relationship has been noted in studies of impramine and amitriptyline, although some studies of amitriptyline suggest a curvilinear form similar to that found for nortriptyline. Studies suggest, though there is as yet insufficient data for confirmation, that the secondary amine TCA doxepin and the tetracyclic antidepressant maprotiline, which has a side chain structure of the secondary amine type, have response-concentration curves of the curvilinear form.

The curves in the preceeding figure represent a compilation or composite of individual curves from the studies of patients. Taking Figure 43 as an example, one patient may have a maximum probability of response at a plasma concentration of 100ng/ml whilst another has this effect at 135ng/ml. Therefore, it is not correct to say that a plasma value within the therapeutic window or above the minimal therapeutic level ensures optimal clinical response to the given TCA. It is still necessary to "titrate" each patient in the step-wise fashion discussed earlier using the clinical symptoms as the definitive criteria of improvement and response. Plasma levels are a guide to therapy but not a "litmus" test or short cut that eliminates clinical examination and assessment.

Before assaying the TCA, it is necessary that sufficient time has elapsed to allow a steady state condition to establish for the TCA between the blood and nervous tissue. In view of the typical plasma half-life of the TCAs, this steady state condition will be achieved in some seven to ten days, and in many cases a day or so earlier. In cases where the plasma half-life is prolonged, for example, in geriatric patients due to aging factors, in patients receiving other medications which influence TCA pharmokinetics or those with specific disease such as hepatic insufficiencies, the steady state for a fixed daily dose of TCA may not be achieved for three or four weeks. The values given in Table 7 are for steady state conditions.

The time elapsed between the last oral dose of the TCA and the drawing of the venous blood sample is important. If the fixed daily dose is being given in divided doses throughout the day, a time lapse of three to seven hours is required before drawing a sample. If the daily dose is given in a single administration, then a delay of twelve or more hours is required for the transient loading peak to diminish and steady state to be reestablished. Clearly, if the patient takes the single dose at bedtime the sample can be appropriately drawn the next morning.

To illustrate the advantages of plasma level determinations as an adjunct to TCA therapy, consider establishing a therapeutic trail of nortriptyline in a geriatric patient with some accompanying hepatic and cardiovascular problems who is also receiving medications for hypertension, hypothyroidism and rheumatoid arthritis (it should be noted that these patients can also have a primary depression).

The stepwise titration of the TCA which was used as an example earlier can be used again. Perhaps, in view of the accompanying problems, one would begin with 50 or 75 milligrams of nortriptyline in a single bedtime dose. The response to this TCA will be assessed on a daily basis and the onset of possible side-effects will be monitored during this time. The decision to shift the dose of the TCA by an increment will be made, typically, in seven days and at this time a plasma sample can be drawn.

Most clinicians can obtain the results of the plasma essay from the laboratory within a couple of days. The result will indicate whether the patient is an abnormal metaboliser of nortriptyline. For example, if the plasma level is 25ng/ml then one has a patient who is a hypermetaboliser of nortriptyline. The chances of them having a clinical response to this dose of nortriptyline is very low. More importantly if one is rigidly "conservative" in prescribing the TCA because of such factors as age or liver disease then in all probability this patient will never get an adequate therapeutic trial of nortriptyline. They will likely be classified as a "therapeutic failure" when in fact it was an unnecessary error resulting in the patient being inadequately treated.

On the other hand, this first plasma level may come back at 200 ng/ml. This warns that the patient is a hypometaboliser of the TCA because of the additional clinical factors and one ought to not increase the dosage of the nortriptyline. In fact, because of the well established curvilinear relationship between the probability for response and plasma concentration for this particular TCA, the step-wise titration of the nortriptyline should be an incremental reduction of the oral dose rather than an increase.

The titration technique for establishing a therapeutic trial of TCAs does not significantly prolong the treatment period and adding plasma level determinations to the protocol does not prolong the drug trial. In fact, identification of a patient's abnormal pharmokinetics some five days into treatment may shorten the overall hospitalisation in the long run. Obviously, the use of plasma levels as a guide to therapy aids in the tailoring of the prescribing to the particular patient and increases the safety factor.

If a patient recovers following a therapeutic trial at a plasma level, for example, of 110ng/ml then this level can serve as a "benchmark" for this TCA. For instance, if they are receiving the TCA on an outpatient basis and need to have other medications prescribed which interfere with the TCA pharmokinetics, then plasma levels allow adjustment of the oral dose of TCA to maintain the level around 110ng/ml.

Periodic determinations of plasma levels during outpatient treatment with a TCA will answer the question of patient compliance which can be a useful piece of information. Just as patients may be inappropriately classified as drug failures in treatment of an acute episode, they may be incorrectly taken to be drug prophylaxis failures in outpatient management when in fact the problem was compliance failure.

3. Monoamine Oxidase Inhibitors (MAOI)

In the early 1950's it was noticed that some patients receiving the antituberculous drug isoniazid showed an improvement in their mood, appetite and initiative. It was later found that isoniazid was a monoamine oxidase inhibitor. The "life cycle" of the principle neurotransmitters was discussed in an earlier chapter. Briefly, these biogenic amines are synthesised from aminoacid precursors in the presynaptic terminal and are released from vesicle storage into the synaptic cleft (Figure 17). The catalytic breakdown of the neurotransmitters occurs in the mitochondria of the presynaptic terminal following active reuptake from the synaptic cleft across the presynaptic membrane (Figure 18).

A principle enzyme involved in this deamination is monoamine oxidase. This is widely distributed in the brain and elsewhere and being particularly located in mitochondrial membrane. Monoamine oxidase is involved in free tyramine, norepinephrine, dopamine, serontonin and other biogenic amines being reduced to inactive metabolites.

It was found that iproniazid, a derivitive of isoniazid, reversed the "depression" induced in animal models by administration of reserpine. This type of information, along with other laboratory and clinical findings, led to iproniazid's introduction in the late 1950's as an antidepressant.

Iproniazid was soon withdrawn from the market as an antidepressant following reports of associated hepatic necrosis in approximately 1 in 5000 of the treated patients. In some cases, the hepatic problems proved to be fatal.

A number of other MAOI's were subsequently developed in order to avoid this liver problem and currently three major groups, namely, *hydrazine, non-hydrazine* and *selective* MAOI drugs are available. Hepatocellular jaundice has been reported in some patients treated with the hydrazine MAOI's but not in those given the non-hydrazine group. Some of the more common MAOI's are given in the following table along with a "typical" daily dosage required for the treatment of major depressive episodes.

The step-wise titration method described for establishing a therapeutic trial of TCA's can be used with the monoamine oxidase inhibitors. The required dose may be given in divided doses through the day or in a single administration. Since the half-life of these medications is

	mg per day
Hydrazine	
phenelzine (Nardil)	45-60
isocarboxazid (Marplan)	45-60
Non-hydrazine	
tranylcypromine (Parnate)	30-40
Selective MAOI	
clorgyline (MAOa)	
deprenyl (MAOb)	

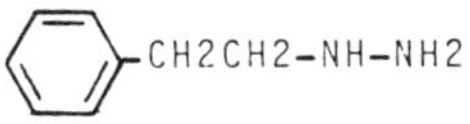

phenelzine

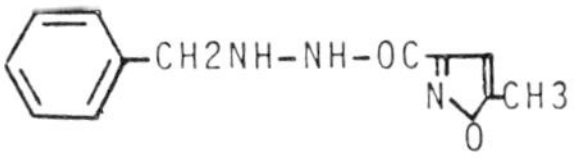

isocarboxazid

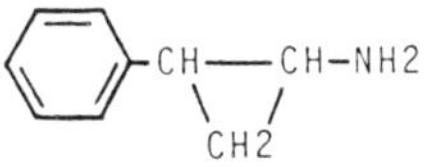

tranylcypromine

Table 8

typically 24 to 36 hours, then a five to seven day interval in adjusting the dosage can be used in the titration. The duration of an adequate trial of TCA's was given as three to four weeks but in the case of the MAOI's this is more likely to be six to eight weeks. As will be mentioned later, the need for a longer therapeutic trial may well be a reflection of the type of depressive syndrome which these drugs are used to treat.

From a clinical viewpoint, the MAOI's have not lived up to the initial expectations as antidepressants. Some controlled studies comparing them to the TCA's suggest that they are equally effective but the majority of studies show them to be inferior to the TCA's. There are no controlled studies of MAOI therapy of primary depression which shows that they are superior to the TCA's.

The current tendency is to use the MAOI's in the treatment of so-called *atypical depression.* A major problem in assessing the effectiveness of the MAOI's is the nature of the symptom profile found in the atypical depressions. A large percentage of the depressive syndromes referred to as atypical depressions show a great deal of situational reactivity, social stresses and problematic personality traits in the presenting symptom profile. At various times, these disorders have been referred to as *neurotic depressions, reactive depressions* or *spectrum depressions.* It may well be that because of this feature a drug trial does not have much of a "fighting chance" when compared to the more endogenous or autonomous disorders such as primary depression.

The MAOI's are currently popular in the treatment of specific variants of atypical depression such as *panic disorders* and *mono-symptomatic phobias.* Just as it is questionable that particular TCA's are specific for certain symptoms of a primary depression, so it is that MAOI's are "syndrome specific." It is worth noting that a number of fundamentally different psychotropic drugs such as benzodiazepines, adrenergic blockers, and TCA's as well as MAOI's have been reported to have success in "particular" disorders such as panic and mono-symptomatic phobias.

The MAOI's should be considered in patients who fail to respond to adequate therapeutic trials of other types of antidepressants. It is highly unlikely that MAOI's would be the first choice in cases of primary depression but there is the possibility that some patients with this disorder would respond having "failed" on therapeutic trials of TCA's.

As one would expect from the mode of action, there is a risk of precipitating a hypertensive episode with MAOI's. The incidence is estimated at some .05 percent with a mortality due to intracranial hemorrhage, of some 0.001 percent.

The selective monoamine oxidase inhibitors, such as clorgyline and deprenyl, are of interest with respect to hypertensive problems. MAO exists in two functionally different forms. Monoamine oxidase type A perferentially deaminates norepinephrine and serotonin. Type B monoamine oxidase preferentially deaminates dopamine and phenylethylamine. It may well be that a selective MAOI can be made with significantly less chance of hypertensive problems.

It is necessary that patients taking MAOI's avoid foods which are rich in vasopressor amines in order to reduce the risk of hypertensive problems. In particular, this refers to food rich in *tyramine* such as yeast products, aged cheese and wine. Care should be taken not to over alarm patients into concluding that a cheeseburger will be lethal.

The onset of a hypertensive episode following ingestion of vasopressor rich food varies from thirty minutes to twenty four hours. Typically the crisis lasts for a couple of hours. A dose of 50 to 100 milligrams of chlorpromazine given intramuscularly will both calm the patient and help the hypertension in most cases. In more serious episodes, 6 milligrams of phentolamine given intravenously will usually be effective. If necessary, the MAOI's can be restarted within twenty four hours of the episode.

It should be noted that MAOI's have a tendency in some patients to significantly lower the blood glucose. This can prove to be a difficult clinical differentiation in patients with prominent anxiety symptoms. Also, these drugs can effectively suppress the REM stages of sleep which sometimes provides a useful alternative to amphetamines in the management of narcolepsy.

As would be expected from their mode of action, there are a wide range of drugs whose effects will be potentiated by MAOI's. For example, meperidine, barbiturates, methyldopa, ganglionic blockers, procaine and chloral hydrate as well as the sympathomimetic agents.

Since monoamine oxidase enzymes are widely distributed throughout the body, there is a wide range of associated side-effects. There occurrence does not necessarily imply toxicity. It will be noted that some of these side-effects do not "fit" the simple model of inhibition of MAO and this indicates the complexity of the neuropharmacology of these drugs. For instance, a frequently associated side-effect of the MAOI's is orthostatic hypotension and dizziness. It should be noted in passing that taking L-tryptophan along with MAOI can significantly increase the serotonin levels and result in a precipitous fall in the patients blood pressure.

Other common side-effects associated with MAOI's include dry mouth, blurring of vision, hesitency with micturation, constipation and some delayed ejaculation.

In cases of serious MAOI overdose, there is a progression of clinical findings as the drug permeates the body. Initially, a few hours after ingestion of the MAOI load, the patient becomes restless, irritable, agitated and hyperactive. Confusion occurs and may quickly progress to a state of coma. In addition to marked hypertension, there is tachypnea, tachycardia, hyperthermia, dilated pupils and increased deep tendon reflexes.

This situation needs careful clinical management. Acidification of the urine will help excretion of the MAOI and in some cases it may be necessary to employ hemodialysis. Careful titration of a neuroleptic to deal with the notably disturbed mental state is invariably required and is preferable to drugs such as benzodiazepines.

4. Second Generation Antidepressants

Since the general introduction of iproniazid and imipramine in the 1960's, a variety of new antidepressants have been developed. Some of these new antidepressants, from a clinical standpoint, are "me too" derivitives of the prototypes with little significant differences in their basic properties. However, some of these new antidepressants, the so-called *second generation,* are fundamentally different from the MAOI and TCA prototypes.

Structurally, as can be seen from the following figure, the commoner second generation drugs differ significantly from the TCA's.

Some of the second generation drugs are reported as having noticeably lower incidences of anticholinergic side-effects which, if confirmed by current studies, will prove to be clinically advantageous. It must be borne in mind that a significant number of patients cannot tolerate prototype TCA's and MAOI's because of these anticholinergic side-effects.

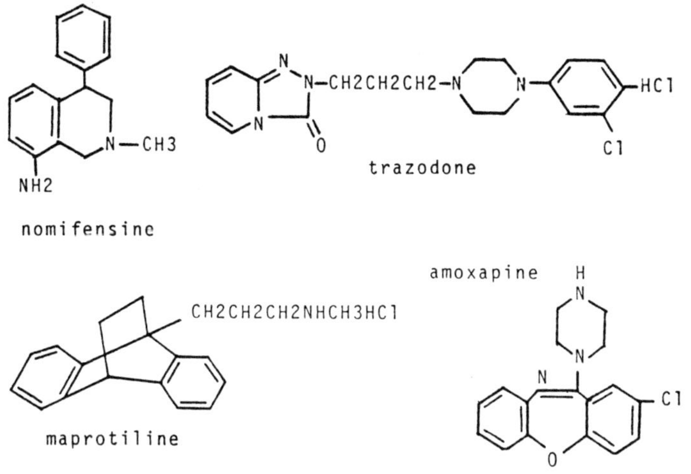

Figure 44

As can be seen from Table 6, some of the second generation drugs have a more specific and selective amine pump blockade. This may account for some of the differences in the central and peripheral side-effects but, more importantly, this neurotransmitter specificity may allow "focusing" on biochemical subtypes of the depressive syndrome which are thought to exist by a number of clinicians and basic scientists.

It was mentioned earlier in this section that amitriptyline has been suggested by some studies to be a preferred TCA in the treatment of depressive syndromes which feature the symptom of insomnia. Whilst the opinion was offered that it is unlikely that a particular TCA would be able to address a specific symptom better than other types of TCA, the fact remains that the antidepressants do have a relative range of sedative properties. The development of sedation in the early phase of treatment is a frequent reason for patients to discontinue their medication. There are advantages in having an antidepressant with a relatively low level of sedation.

The following table ranks the initial sedative effects of some antidepressants. It must be remembered that patient idiosyncracies, regarding pharmacology play an important role in these side-effects. Some of the second generation antidepressants are said to have very low sedative properties which could prove to be very advantageous.

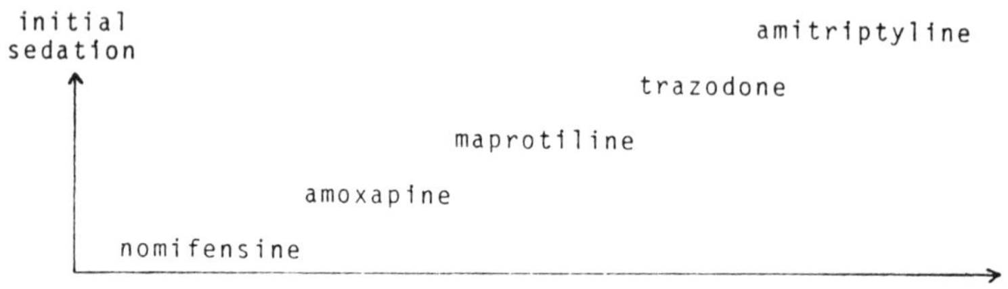

Table 9

i. Amoxapine

This antidepressant has a structure with features of the prototype TCA imipramine and the neuroleptic loxapine. Specifically, it is the demethylated metabolite of loxapine, tricyclic dibenzoxazepine.

Studies of amoxapine indicate an effectiveness of the treatment of depressive syndromes comparable to first generation TCA's. However, some studies are lacking in terms of a "tight" design concerning placebo controls and patient selection. It has been suggested that this antidepressant has a faster onset of action than prototype TCA's but this may well be due to some of its neuroleptic activity, for example, associated anxiolytic and sedative properties. This claim to have a faster antidepressant effect onset needs further confirmation since the fact that a drug is rapidly absorbed and quickly reaches steady state conditions need not mean a correspondingly quicker effect.

It should be noted that amoxapine, because of its neuroleptic characteristics, may have a higher incidence of extrapyramidal side-effects. Akasthesia has been reported and it will be interesting to see in the future the number of reports of tardive dyskinesia like syndromes.

The typical daily dose for a therapeutic trial is 200 to 300 milligrams per day. Amoxapine has a plasma half life of some 8 hours and its active metabolite 8-hydroxy-amoxapine has a half life of some 24 hours. This combination allows administration of the daily requirement in a single dose and establishment of steady state within five to seven days.

It does not follow that since amoxapine has tricyclic and neuroleptic structural features it would be specifically indicated in the treatment of "psychotic" depression nor in "depressed" schizophrenics. These points were discussed earlier in the text. However, it should be noted that amoxapine does not fall under the heading of the combination psychotropic medications such as Triavil.

ii. Maprotiline

This is a tetracyclic agent. The structure, n-alkol-substituted dibenzodicyclo octadienes, bears a similarity to the secondary TCA's. The main difference is a "fourth" ring formed over the central tricyclic ring by a dimethyl bridge.

This drug's side-effect profile is basically equivalent in terms of type and incidence to that of the prototype TCA's. Perhaps one point of clinical significance is the incidence of seizures. All antidepressants will lower the seizure threshold to some degree and it is unlikely that maprotiline is more prone to induce seizures than other antidepresants. However, seizures are reported to be dose related and begin with relatively low daily oral doses of maprotiline.

The "typical" required daily dose for a therapeutic effect is 150 to 300 milligrams. Studies indicate that this tetracyclic is as effective as TCA's in the treatment of primary depressive disorders. It is said maprotiline shows a quicker therapeutic effect than prototype TCA's during the second week of treatment. However, this difference is not apparent by the third week of treatment. It remains questionable as to whether or not maprotiline has a fster overall onset of effect than the prototype TCA's. The tetracyclic does reach its peak plasma level some eight hours following oral administration but this does not necessarily mean that it "kicks in" at this point. The steady state conditions for a fixed daily dose are established in some seven to ten days akin to the prototype TCA's since the plasma half-life of this drug is similar to that of the TCA's.

iii. Trazodone

This is a phenylpiperazine derivitive of trizolopyridine. As can be seen from Figure 44, the structure has features similar to those found in the indolamine neurotransmitter serotonin.

Trazodone inhibits the presynaptic reuptake of serotonin while having little effect on the reuptake of norepinephrine. This feature of biogenic amine selectivity is perhaps the major feature of this second generation antidepressant. Even though its serotonin blockade is weaker than some of the prototype TCA's, this is compensated for by the selectivity factor.

Also, it has low muscarinic receptor affinity which results in a decreased incidence of anticholingergic side-effects. In addition, it has central alpha-adrenergic blockade properties which likely increases catecholamine turnover.

The relatively low incidence of anticholinergic side-effects compared to TCA's is useful in patients who find such prevent continuation of treatment. Although laboratory studies show the antimuscarinic effects to be very low, the incidence of the clinical anticholinergic side-effects is not equally reduced. This is another example of the unfortunate truth that many laboratory findings do not "travel well" to the bedside.

The selectivity of reuptake blockade and central adrenergic blockade along with low antimuscarinic effects suggests that trazodone would have notably less cardiovascular side-effects than the prototype antidepressants. There is a definite need for more clinical data in this regard. Initially, trazodone was felt to be low in terms of inducing cardiac changes but more recently there has been a need to reconsider this point.

This antidepressant has a "typical" commencement dose of 100 to 200 milligrams daily. It may be necessary to titrate this to 500 or 600 milligrams in some patients for the desired therapeutic responce. Therapeutic trials indicate that trazodone is as effective as the prototype TCA's in the treatment of primary depressive disorders.

iv. Nomifensine

This is a tetrahydroisoquinoline antidepressant. It has weak reuptake inhibition of serotonin but effectively blocks reuptake of norepinephine and dopamine at the pre-synaptic terminal. Nomifensine has the additional property of dopamine reuptake blockade at central synapses.

A feature of this antidepressant is the low incidence of cardiovascular side-effects. As stressed earlier, side-effects involving the cardiovascular system are frequently important in the choice of an antidepressant. The orthostatic hypotensive effects of nomifensine are minimal compared to the prototype TCA's. At therapeutic doses, nomifensine does not produce cardiac abnormalities and the lethal cardiotoxic effects seen with TCA overdoses are not reported on suicide attempts with this medication. Studies suggest that this antidepressant has a relatively low incidence of sedation at therapeutic doses.

The plasma half life of nomifensine is some two hours so that the required daily dose cannot be given as a single administration. Studies suggest that the required daily dose for a therapeutic effect is between 75 and 200 milligrams. Clinical trials indicate that this antidepressant is comparable with the prototype TCA's, however, there is a clear need for more controlled studies, in particular those involving hospitalised patients with primary depressive disorders.

5. Lithium

This is a monovalent cation which places close to sodium and potassium on the periodic table. The modern use of lithium in the treatment of some functional psychoses stems from the work of Cade. He was interested in a possible relationship between the urea cycle and behavioral disorders in laboratory animals, in particular the "manic" type. Cade used lithium urate in these studies and came to the conclusion that the important components which influenced the "manic" animals behaviour was not the urea but rather the lithium.

Cade published his work in the late 1940's but lithium as an agent to treat mania was not generally available in the United States until the late 1960's. An important factor in the delay was problems with the earlier use of lithium as a salt substitute in the management of hypertension. It is also said, with a deal of truth, that the pharmaceutical companies did not press lithium's introduction since, being a natural salt, it could not be patented.

Usually, lithium is given to the patient in the form of lithium carbonate. The capsule form tends to have a better absorption coefficient than the tablet preparation and the capsule causes less gastrointestinal upset than does the tablet. The difference in absorption of these two preparations should be taken into account if a patient switches from capsule to tablet or vice versa. The capsule and tablet contain 300 milligrams of lithium carbonate which comprises 8 milliequivalents of element lithium.

Absorption from the GI tract into the blood stream occurs in some four to six hours after which lithium is distributed throughout the body in relation to water. There is a significant delay in lithium's crossing of the blood brain barrier and establishing of steady state conditions within the central nervous system. This delay, some three to seven days, means that despite "therapeutic" plasma levels there will be little to no clinical effects of lithium during this time.

This delay in the onset of a clinical response due to lithium's "inertia" in crossing the blood brain barrier can be a significant factor in the initial phase of treatment of a manic patient. Similarly, there is a delay in the clearance of lithium from the central nervous system. In the course of a lithium washout, the plasma level may be reported as zero but clinical evidence of some lithium still present in the nervous system may be apparent.

Since lithium, following body fluids, enters most organs, and patients are often maintained on this medication for months and years, it is imperative that an adequate workup is done before prescribing this medication. The important elements of a pre-lithium work-up are as follows.

i. Renal Function

This is the critical organ for evaluation since over 95 percent of lithium is excreted via the kidneys. At this point, it is helpful to outline a simplified model of kidney function as it applies to lithium. This is shown schematically in the following figure.

Sodium is actively reabsorbed in the proximal tubule by a carrier limited process. Lithium is reabsorbed by the same process and therefore is in direct competition with sodium.

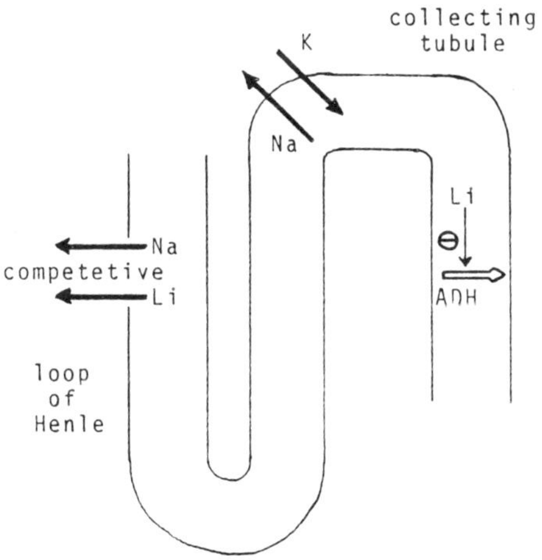

Figure 45

The sodium which is not reabsorbed in the proximal tubule will present at the distal tubule where some will be reabsorbed in exchange for potassium. Some of the lithium which is not reabsorbed in the proximal tubule presents in the distal tubule where it inhibits the action of antidiuretic hormone (ADH).

Therefore, if no alteration is sodium and potassium intake occurs, a patient begun on lithium therapy may over time become potassium depleted because of the increased presentation of sodium at the distal tubules. This tendency of lithium to produce hypokalemia can be a crucial point during prolonged lithium therapy. It is likely to have been a factor in the problems of lithium being prescribed as a salt substitute in hypertension management.

Patients receiving lithium whose sodium intake is subsequently decreased are in danger of becoming lithium toxic. Those whose sodium intake is increased while receiving a fixed lithium dose will have a reduction in their plasma lithium levels. The lithium treated patient who is begun on a salt-wasting diuretic needs to have a reduction in their lithium intake otherwise they may, over time, become lithium toxic.

The prefered work-up of renal function involves a 24 hour urine collection for determination of creatinine clearance. It is not sufficient to determine a patient's serum creatinine and blood urea nitrogen since under various circumstances these spot values can be normal despite compromised renal function. From the same 24 hour unine collection, the daily protein excretion can be determined which can be an important benchmark in the monitoring of patients on long-term lithium maintainence.

It is often impossible to collect a 24 hour urine from a patient with acute mania. An estimate of the renal status can be obtained from the serum creatinine and blood urea nitrogen. A method of estimating the required lithium dosage and in addition giving an indication of the acute manic's renal clearance of lithium can be obtained from a loading procedure which is shown in Figure 46 and will be discussed in detail later in this chapter.

ii. Blood Panel (SMAC)

The multichannel blood analysis will include serum creatine and blood urea nitrogen as well as liver enzymes, protein and blood glucose. Also included on this panel are the serum electrolytes. Clearly, one needs to be aware of the sodium, potassium, chloride and bicarbonate levels prior to beginning lithium.

iii. Hematology Changes

Lithium produces a leukocytosis in most patients and a white cell count of 12 to 14 thousand is not unusual. It is important to note the prelithium cell count so that increases are not incorrectly ascribed to infection. The lithium induced leukocytosis does not have the shift of cells one sees in response to an infection, rather it consists predominantly of mature white cells.

Studies show that these mature cells have not been mobilised from the marginated cells of the vascular system but are derived directly from the bone marrow. The implication is that lithium has a direct stimulation effect on bone marrow stem cells. This has lead to the use of lithium in patients who have dysplastic bone marrow and it has proved to be effective in some cases.

iv. Thyroid Function

Lithium has an inhibitory effect on thyroid function. A simple model for this effect is that lithium incorporates into the sodium-potassium pump in place of sodium and alters membrane transport. This substitution produces the "inertia" of blood brain barrier transport mentioned earlier and influences transport across other membranes such as that in the thyroid gland.

The thyroid gland uptake of iodine is impaired by lithium as is the release of thyroid hormone across the thyroid membrane into the blood stream. Lithium also impairs the coupling of iodotyrosine in the manufacture of thyroid hormones.

Initiation of lithium therapy results in a slight suppression of thyroid function. In the majority of cases, this is rapidly corrected by a slight increase in thyroid stimulating hormone (TSH) and accompanying increase of the thyroid gland's output. However, if the person's thyroid status is precarious, then lithium therapy may prove to be problematic.

A patient may be euthyroid only because of a sustained high level of TSH and/or thyroid cells which are functioning at their upper limit. Initiation of lithium and its resulting thyroid suppression may not be able to be compensated for by a further increase in TSH and/or increase in thyroid cell output.

This state of precarious euthyroidism would not have been recognised if the prelithium screening of thyroid function had been limited to serium T4, T3 resin uptake and free thyroxine index determinations. A better indication would have been given if, in addition to these tests, a serum TSH value had been obtained. For patients who are expected to be on chronic lithium maintainence, all four thyroid function tests are advisable. The TSH value is a useful check during chronic treatment with lithium since it indicates the "reserve" of the pituitary-thyroid axis in maintaining euthyroidism.

Some ten percent of patients receiving lithium therapy will develop a goiterous nodule. The problem will resolve with discontinuation of the lithium and there have been no reports of these nodules becoming malignant. Often the clinical situation does not allow for discontinuation of lithium. If a patient is driven hypothyroid by lithium therapy, this can be simple corrected by thyroid replacement. In passing it should be mentioned that lithium can influence carbohydrate metabolism. The glucose tolerance curves may show a slight elevation but this is rarely of clinical significance.

v. Cardiovascular System

As would be expected from the simple sodium-potassium membrane pump model, lithium incorporates in the myocardium and interferes with intracardiac conduction and cardiac contractility. A base-line EKG is important in the prelithium evaluation.

There may be prolongation of conduction times involving PR, QRS and QT intervals and some ST-T segment changes on the electrocardiogram. Lithiuum rarely produces clinically significant changes in the cardiovascular system at therapeutic or non-toxic levels.

vi. Pregnancy

It is important to be aware of the possible teratogenic effects of all medications. Lithium is frequently prescribed for patients in the childbearing age group. It crosses the placenta and is present in the breast milk of mothers.

An increase in congenital cardiac abnormalities has been reported in association with lithium treatment. It is a matter of clinical judgement whether lithium shoud be discontinued during the first trimester of pregnancy since a reoccurrence of a primary affective illness could have serious repercussions for the mother and her unborn child.

Following the prelithium workup, it is necessary to quickly establish a therapeutic level of lithium in the patient. Typically, this requires administration of 300 miligrams three or four times per day. The fact that lithium is absorbed, "used" and excreted as lithium means that it does not have the complex pharmokinetics associated with such psychotropic agents as the neuroleptics and antidepressants. However, there are patient idiosyncracies which require the "tailoring" of the lithium to each patient.

In using plasma level determinations to aid in the prescribing of lithium, it is necessary that some points are understood. Firstly, the plasma level is used to indicate the concentration of lithium within the central nervus system since the latter cannot be measured in clinical practise. The plasma level gives this information only after sufficient time has elapsed to allow the plasma and central nervous system to have equilibriated.

The fact that it takes some four days, and in some cases up to three times as long, for lithium to cross the blood brain barrier means that drawing venous blood for determination of therapeutic levels requires this length of time on a fixed daily dose before sampling. If samples are drawn sooner, one is in fact generating a "loading" curve for the medication in the patient. Secondly, since lithium is rapidly absorbed into the blood stream it would be pointless to draw a sample for plasma assay within a few hours of the patient taking an oral dose of lithium. An ideal time for sampling is prior to the day's first dose of lithium.

One method of beginning lithium therapy is shown schematically in the following figure. It has a number of clinical advantages.

Day 1 has the administration of 600 milligrams of lithium carbonate, two capsules, in a single dose at 7:00 am. No additional lithium is given that day. At 7:00 am on Day 2, a venous blood sample is drawn and sent to the laboratory for a plasma-lithium determination. Clearly, this is neither a steady state determination nor does it meaningfully reflect the central nervous system status but rather is a single point on this patients lithium loading curve.

Following the drawing of the blood sample on Day 2, the patient is begun on 300 milligrams of lithium three times per day. Prior to the third dose, the plasma level of lithium should be available from the laboratory. This plasma value can then be read against the following nomogram.

Plasma lithium 24 hours after a 600mg dose (meq/litre)	Approx daily dose for steady state to be in the therapeutic window
less than 0.05	1200 mg tid
0.05/0.09	900 mg tid
0.10/0.14	600 mg tid
0.15/0.19	300 mg qid
0.20/0.23	300 mg tid
0.24/0.30	300 mg bid
more than 0.30	300 mg bid (with caution)

Table 10

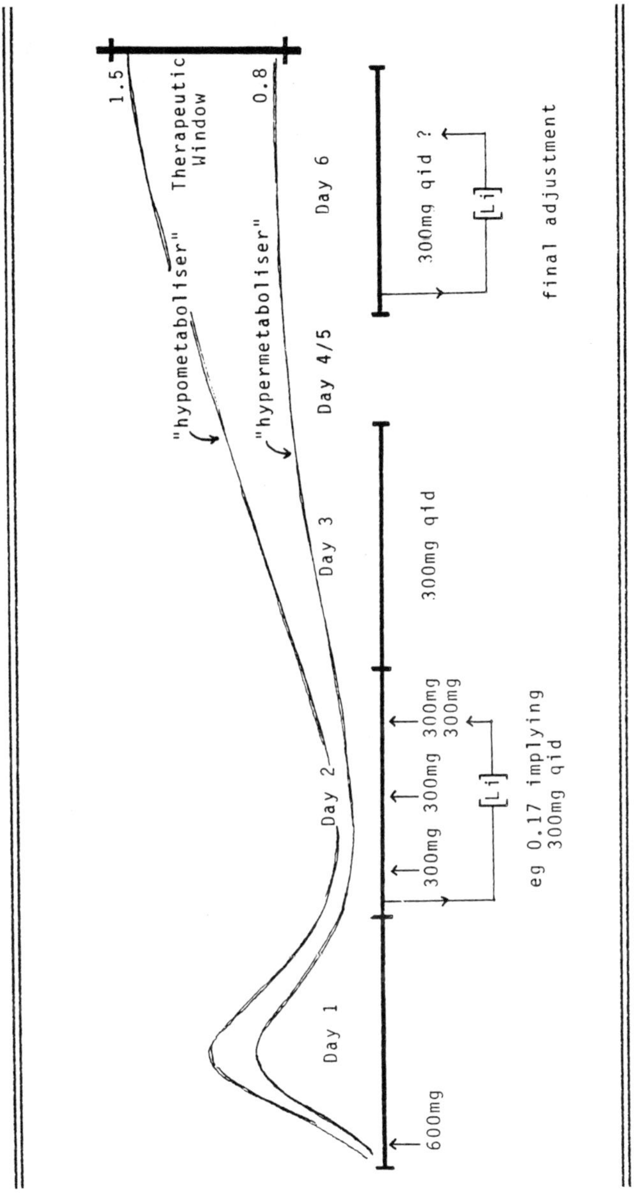
1.5
Therapeutic Window
0.8
"hypometaboliser"
"hypermetaboliser"
Day 1
Day 2
Day 3
Day 4/5
Day 6
600mg
300mg 300mg 300mg 300mg
[Li]
eg 0.17 implying 300mg qid
300mg qid
300mg qid ?
[Li]
final adjustment

Figure 46

One of the reasons that a simple nomogram can be constructed for lithium as opposed, for example, to the TCA's or neuroleptics is that lithium has less patient idiosyncracies in pharmokinetics. A correction by either adding to the day's third dose of lithium or withholding it depends on the dosage given on this nomogram. If the nomogram suggests 300 milligrams four times per day, then on Day 3, 4 and 5 the patient receives that dose and the evening dose on the second day consists of 600 milligrams. A suggested dose of 300 milligrams twice per dcay results in the evening dose of Day 2 being withheld and then 300 milligrams twice per day on Days 3, 4 and 5.

It must be stressed that the dosage predicted from the nomogram is not the definitive daily requirement to put the patient into the therapeutic range. It is an approximation which succeeds in avoiding extreme errors due to idiosyncratic retention or elimination of lithium. In many cases, it is necessary to make a final adjustment in the lithum dose.

A particular advantage of this 600 milligram loading dose technique is that it gives some indication of lithium's renal clearance. A high 24 hour plasma level raises the possibility of impaired renal function and suggests caution. The definitive 24 hour urine collection to determine the patient's creatinine clearance can be done later when the patient is calmer.

On Day 6, a blood sample is drawn prior to the day's first dose of lithium. Since the plasma half life of lithium is typically 24 hours, this sample should indicate the steady state lithium level and reflect an equilibrium state between blood and brain tissue. A final adjustment in the oral lithium dosage based on this result can then be made to bring the patient into the *therapeutic range.*

The therapeutic range of lithium is well established from numerous controlled clinical studies. These studies show that for the treatment of acute mania, the steady state plasma level of lithium should be in range 0.8 to 1.5 *milliequivalents per liter.* In severe mania, it is well to have the patient in the upper portion of this therapeutic range.

Often, as the manic episode resolves, those patients running at 1.5 milliequivalents per liter can be adequately controlled in the lower reaches of the "window." Therefore once again, as in the case of the TCA's and neuroleptics, it is necessary to *titrate* the medication against the clinical symptoms for each patient.

The therapeutic range of lithium as a prophylactic medication in the primary affective disorder is wider than that for acute mania. This is to be expected given the symptoms and natural course of these disorders. Studies indicate that the prophylactic range is 0.5 to 1.5 *miliequivalents per liter.* The question of prophylaxis will be discussed in more detail later in the text.

Lithium therapy has a range of associated side-effects and there is patient idiosyncracy in terms of their occurrence and severity. These side-effects can be divided into three groups. Those of Group 1 occur at plasma levels within the therapeutic and prophylactic ranges. They are not related to lithium toxicity and invariably do not require alterations in the lithum dosage. In some cases, they will remit after a few days or weeks but should they continue the symptoms are minimal compared to these of this major affective disorder.

i. Group 1, Tremor

This is a fine tremor which usually involves the hands. It is both an at-rest and action tremor that is often difficult to differentiate from anxiety. In most cases, the tremor is not too problematic but if, for example, the patient is a draughtsman or surgeon it can be debilitating. The beta-blocker propranolol is very useful in the management of this side-effect. It can be titrated against the symptoms and typically 20 to 40 milligrams orally per day is effective.

ii. Group I, Nausea/GI Upset

Many patients have gastrointestinal upset due to taking lithium. Usually, this occurs after swallowing the capsule and lasts for some 30 minutes but for some patients it lasts throughout the day. Lithobid is a slow release preparation of lithium which avoids the peaking of blood lithium and lessens the nausea. In a few patients, changing the lithium preparation from the usual bicarbonate to a sulphate or chloride may reduce idiosyncratic gastrointestinal difficulties.

iii. Group I, Malaise/Dizziness/Fatigue

Malaise may well be a reflection of the gastrointestinal upset as could be the dizziness and fatigure. There are times, as in the case of the side-effects of the TCA's, when it is difficult to decide whether complaints are drug related or symptomatic of the major affective disorder. Dizziness may be reported as vertigo but usually it lacks the rotational features associated with the classical Meniere's syndrome.

iv. Group 1, Polyuria Polydipsia

This is an important Group 1 side-effect since its being misunderstood can lead to lithium toxicity.

After a few days or weeks on a therapeutic dose of lithium a patient can develop polyuria-polydipsia. In many cases, this is inconvenient rather than problematic. However, if it continues to increase, and if the patient is a truckdriver or steeplejack, it can become debilitating. Although the patient is not lithium toxic, it is desirable to lessen the side-effect if possible while keeping the lithium at the required level.

A common mistake is to conclude that since intake and excretion of fluid has increased then "lithium is being washed out at a greater rate" and so "an increase in lithium dosage is required to maintain the earlier therapeutic plasma level." This is not true. If the oral dose of lithium is increased, then over a period of months the patient will be driven lithium toxic. Also, an increase in dosage can make the polyuria-polydipsa worse and lead to further incorrect increases in the administered lithium.

The fact that there is an increase in the amount of fluid moved through the kidney does not mean that lithium, sodium or potassium will be "pulled" from the nephron's wall and thereby flushed down the tubule. The grand design of the kidney would be lacking if this were true since it would mean that three extra pints, with equivalent urination, could lead to serious electrolyte imbalances.

Also, it must be noted that this polyuria-polydipsia is not due to the onset of diabetes insipidus. There has been no sudden decrease in the patients production of antidiuretic hormone (ADH). Administration of ADH will have no discernible effect on the problem.

The polyuria-polydipsia is a nephrogenic diabetes insipidus due to lithum's inhibition of the action of ADH at the receptor level in the distal tubule. This is schematically shown in Figure 45. Clearly, reduction of the lithium dose will reduce the side-effect but the patient will likely have a relapse of the major affective disorder.

Some 10 to 20 percent of patients obtain a reduction in the polyuria-polydipsia with the administration of the diuretic hydrochlorothiazide. Administration of a diuretic to treat diuresis may at first sight seem paradoxical. The diuretic produces a preferential reabsorption of lithium in comparison to sodium prior to the distal tubule which results in less lithium presenting in the distal nephron to inhibit the action of ADH. This reduction in the lithium inhibition is achieved while still maintaining a therapeutic plasma lithium level. In fact, the plasma lithium level may increase slightly with the addition of hydrochlorothiazide and a reduction in the oral lithium dose may be required to keep the patient's level at its optimum clinical level.

The side-effects of Group 2 are indicative of early lithium toxicity. In general, toxicity begins at lithium plasma levels of 2.0 milliequivalents per litre. The half life of lithium is some 24 hours so discontinuing the medication will correct the problem in most cases within a day or two. The patient can then be seen in the office the day after discontinuing the medication and a plasma level determination will allow a calculation of the previous day's problematic level. It is then necessary to look into the possible causes of the lithium toxicity. In many cases, the problem involves compliance, the recent addition of other medications and diet changes but one must not overlook possible renal difficulties and disorders which are unrelated to lithium per se.

The Group 2 toxicity features drowsiness and somnelence. The patient becomes ataxic and unsteady in their gait in contrast to the fatigue and weakness of Group 1. They also begin to complain of blurred vision.

The signs and symptoms of Group 3 imply severe lithium toxicity. This condition requires hospitalisation. It is an emergency and the patient should not be instructed to stop their medication and come by the office the next day.

i. Group 3, Acute Organic Brain Syndrome

The lithium toxicity results in an acute organic brain syndrome. There is a primary alteration in the level of consciousness with confusion and disorientation. This metabolic brain syndrome can have perturbations of percention, cognition, affect, mobility and behaviour constituting an organic psychosis.

ii. Group 3, Gastrointestinal Tract

The problems at this stage are vomiting and diarrhea rather than nausea and gastric upset. These features can further complicate the fluid and electrolyte problems associated with severe lithium toxicity.

iii. Group 3, Nervous System

Lithium will incorporate in both the central and peripheral nervous system. The delay in entering and leaving the nervous system means that these Group 3 features of lithium toxicity will likely persist for many days. Myoclonic and generalised seizures can occur and lead to coma states. The blurred vision problem of Group 2 is now compounded by nystagmus and possible occular gyric crisis.

It should be noted that although this is a metabolic toxicity, and likely to "diffusely" involve the nervous system to varying degrees, focal abnormalities can occur. For instance, the EEG usually shows a diffuse abnormality but on occasion a focal change is seen which should not be confused with a space-occupying lesion. Similarly, in the peripheral nervous system, lithium toxicity can give rise to asymmetrically neuropathies and increased deep tendon reflexes although symmetrical polyneuropathies are more the case.

The management of Group 3 lithium toxicity is a medical emergency. A key factor in the management is supporting the renal excretion of lithium. This requires careful monitoring of a number of systems including the cardiovascular and pulmonary along with renal fluid and electrolyte problems.

It was pointed out earlier that polyuria-polydipsia did not "flush" out lithium to any significant degree. Therefore, by the same token, fluid loading the lithium toxic patient is not going to significantly increase lithium excretion. Clearly, one gives intravenous fluids, monitors input and out and ensures that the kidney excretes the lithium load but this does not require fluid in the range of 5 or 8 liters per day.

If the renal function is impaired, a diuretic will be of ssistance in maintaining adequate renal output. The preferred diuretic would be of the osmotic variety such as urea, mannitol or aminophyline. These will "pull" out equivalent amounts of lithium and sodium thereby making the electrolyte stability easier to maintain.

Hemodialysis is not without complications but if the patient's renal function is severely impaired it may be a necessary addition in the clinical management. It should be noted that dialysis clears the blood stream but does not directly alter the tissue content of the toxic material. Certainly, reducing the plasma lithium level will increase lithium transport from critical areas such as the nervous system, however, lithium migration from the central nervous system via a concentration gradient is not particularly effective. When it comes to crossing membranes such as the blood-brain-barrier, lithium shows an "inertia" which is troublesome from a number of viewpoints. Hemodialysis certainly has a place in management but it should be reserved for critical cases.

Lithium has a number of clinical applications which will be discussed in the following text.

a. Acute mania

There have been numerous controlled clinical studies demonstrating the effectiveness of lithium in the treatment of acute mania. These studies indicate success rates in the 80 percent range and make this disorder the most established indication for lithium treatment.

There is a significant delay in the onset of action of lithium and its maximum effect may not be seen for some ten days to two weeks. The therapeutic window of 0.8 to 1.5 milliequivalents per liter is well established and should be used as a guide in the titration of lithium against the clinical symptoms.

The neuroleptics will produce amelioration of manic symptoms faster than lithium but they can have side-effects such as sedation and extrapyramidal symptoms. In many cases, the sedative properties of a neuroleptic such as chlorpromazine can be a distinct advantage. It is particularly notable from the clinical studies that lithum "focuses" in on the core symptoms of the mania and has a much more selective and specific "antimanic" effect than the neuroleptics.

In many cases, the clinical situation requires immediacy of action and neuroleptics must be given in conjunction with the lithium. There have been reports of problematic interactions between lithium and neuroleptics, in particular haloperidol. The clinical picture is similar to the neuroleptic malignant syndrome and features hyperpyrexia, mutism, rigidity and later tardive dysknesia. Studies suggest that lithium enhances neuroleptic blocking effects and that phenothiazines tend to increase intracellular lithium levels. These reactions are very rare but the possibility of such occurrences should be borne in mind with combined therapy. Once the lithium level has been established, the neuroleptic can be titrated from the treatment protocol.

b. Prophylaxis of Primary Affective Disorders

The bipolar and unipolar affective disorders have natural courses which are characterised by spontaneous relapses and remissions. During the remission periods, the patients essentially are symptom free and return to a premorbid level of functioning. For such disorders, care should be taken in the definition and use of the word prophylaxis.

The word is used in the sense that relapses which require clinical intervention such as hospitalisation are lessened if the person continues with lithium therapy. However, it should be borne in mind that for long periods of lithum prophylaxis the disorder is "spontaneously" in remission. This presents a common problem in clinical management since some patients discontinue lithium and since they do not relapse for many months conclude that they "do not and never did need lithium therapy."

Controlled clinical trials show that lithium is prophylactic in preventing relapses and/or "muting" the symptom severity of relapses so that rehospitalisation is not required. Lithium is most obviously prophylactic in the *bipolar type* of primary affective disorder. This is true for both the manic and depressive phases of the bipolar illness. The immediate question raised is whether or not this means that lithium is an antidepressant? In the context that prophylaxis was earlier defined, it does not necessarily follow that lithium has specific antidepressant properties because it is prophylactic for the depressive phase. Clearly, controlled studies demonstrate lithium's antimanic affects but at present these are insufficient studies to confirm a specific antidepressant effect.

If a patient receiving lithium prophylaxis begins to show the clinical features of mania, the lithium level should be determined. It may well be that the patient has not complied with the prescribed lithium treatment. The lithium level may be, for example, 0.6 milliequivalents per liter which is within the therapeutic range for prophylaxis but not sufficient for treatment of a manic episode. Clearly, the lithium level should be raised and perhaps it will be necessary to titrate to the upper part of the windout in order to control the symptoms. If clinically necessary, a neuroleptic can be added to the lithium and then titrated out at a later date.

If a lithium prophylaxed patient begins to show the clinical features of depression, then the lithium level should be checked and necessary changes made. It will likely be necessary to add an antidepressant to the lithium for an adequate therapeutic trial. In neither situation should the lithium be discontinued when the other drug, neuroleptic or TCA, is added to the treatment.

There is recent evidence that the response of a primary depression to a TCA can be increased in some instances by the addition of lithium to the pharmacotherapy. This procedure may well be worth considering when a patient has an inadequate response to a therapeutic trial of TCA's.

The evidence that lithium is prophylactic in the *unipolar type* of primary affective disorder is not as strong as in the case of the bipolar type. Some studies indicate that prophylaxis is equally effective using prolonged TCA therapy as using lithium.

However, as was pointed out in an earlier section, some 10 to 20 percent of bipolar patients have their first three episodes of the depressive type and mania does not present until the third relapse. A patient with two depressive episodes may be a bipolar patient and if so could do better with lithium than TCA prophylactic.

The decision to begin litium prophylaxis, both in bipolar and unipolar disorders, is a clinical judgment which depends on a number of factors. Clearly, the more relapses and the more severe they are from a clinical standpoint then the more indication for lithium prophylaxis. The occurrence of mania, and hence the verification of a bipolar illness, will invariably lead to a period of lithium prophylaxis. In the case of unipolar disorders, more than two relapses will lead many clinicians to begin a period of lithium prophylaxis.

The duration of prophylaxis is also a matter of clinical judgement. The decisions are based on the same considerations of neuroleptic prophylaxis of the schizophrenias, namely, that the patient first establishes psycho-social stability and then the medication is titrated down with reference to the patient's functioning and re-emergence of the clinical symptomatology.

Some patients, because of the nature of their illness, have to be maintained on lithium for years, and in some instances decades. This leads to the question of the repercussions of prolonged lithium therapy. This point focuses on the issue of induced renal damage. Early studies suggested that chronic use of lithium over a period of years shows a significant increase in renal damage. This was an irreversible amyloid-like damage located in the distal portion of the nephron. Recent controlled studies, were an adequate prelithium workup of kidney function was done and careful monitoring of kidney function and lithium levels was carried out through years of treatment, shows that renal complications are not significantly increased with chronic lithium administration.

It is important that periodically during lithium prophylaxis evaluation are made of the patient's status. Plasma lithium levels and serum electrolytes should be checked weekly a few times following discharge from the hospital. This checks the patient's ability to comply in the home and work setting. The intervals between these checks can be increased as the prophylaxis continues. Perhaps every six months the thyroid function should be screen. It was mentioned earlier that perhaps a TSH level is the most helpful single parameter to screen for lithium induced changes of the thyroid gland. Once a year, it is prudent to have the patient collect a 24 hour unine. This can be done as an outpatient, to determine protein excretion and creatinine clearance.

Lithium has a place in the treatment of cyclothymic disorders and some particular personality disorders such as *hypomania* and the *emotionally unstable character disorders.* A simple rational to running a therapeutic trial for such disorders is that they may be, as was discussed in an earlier section of the text, "muted" expressions of a primary affective disorder and if so lithium may prove to be a valuable therapy. For example, a hypomanic or cyclothymic personality disorder patient with a positive family history of bipolar illness would suggest a therapeutic trial of lithium. Although controlled studies are limited, partly because of the problems in designing and carrying through studies on such patients, the clinical evidence of successful trials is sufficient to require their consideration.

It is unfortunate that lithium has become something of a "fad" with some clinicians and many of the public. It has the appeal of being a "natural" medication rather than a man-made drug and since affective disorders can feature such an array of accompanying problems it seems to have been proposed in recent years for the treatment of almost every disorder known to man. One disorder of note is its use in the treatment of headaches. Obviously, the non-specific headache may be related to an underlying affective disorder and this is the reason that it is effective. However, the specific example of *cluster headaches* or *histamine headaches,* seems to show a significant response to lithium therapy in the absence of indications of a primary affective disorder. The required plasma level for response is one within the manic therapeutic window.

The mode of action of lithium is unclear at the present time. The main theories focus on the biogenic amine hypotheses of the major affective disorders. In terms of the biogenic amine norepinephrine, the mania properties hinge on a reduction in its availability at the post synaptic receptor. This is supported by experiments which show that lithium increases noreprinephrine reuptake into nerve endings. Studies have shown that in manic patients with elevated MHPG levels, lithium administration will decrease the levels of the norepinephrine metabolite. Other studies indicate that lithium promotes the release of norepinephrine within the neuronal terminal without an increase in the biogenic amines synthesis while decreasing the direct release of noreprinephrine from the nerve terminal.

Lithium has been shown to increase neuronal uptake of the serotonin precursor tryptophan. Also, lithium has been shown to increase the synthesis of serotonin and the formation of its principle metabolite 5HIAA. The proposal is that such adjustment of indolamines helps to "reset" the biogenic amines to restore equilibrium of function. Obviously lithium will influence the bodys electrolyte profile via the so-called sodium-potassium pump, and alteration in membrane and cellular transport. What influence this has on the limbic system and the hypothalamic-pituitary-adrenal axis is presently unknown.

The impact of lithium on clinical practise has been enormous. An estimate of this in dollars was done by looking at patients with a series of major affective episodes who then responded to lithium treatment and prophylaxis. The money saved in hospital costs and productivity were conservatively estimated to be in the billions of dollars over the ensuing decade. What the savings would be if one also included patients who should have had lithium therapy but were denied one can only guess.

REFERENCES

1. Fish's Clinical Psychopathology. Edited by Max Hamilton, John Wright and Sons Ltd., Bristol, United Kingdom, 1981
2. Fish's Schizophrenia. Edited by Max Hamilton, John Wright and Sons Ltd., Bristol, United Kingdom, 1984
3. Psychopathology. By F. Kraupl Taylor. Butterworth and Company Ltd., London, United Kingdom, 1966
4. Cerebral Basis of Psychopathology. By Pierre Flor-Henry, John Wright and Sons Ltd., Bristol, United Kingdom, 1983
5. Neuropharmacology of the Central Nervous System and Behavioural Disorders. Edited by Gene C. Palmer; Academic Press Inc., London, United Kingdom, 1981
6. Clinical Psychiatry. By Eliot Slater and Martin Roth Bailliere, Tindall and Cassell, London, United Kingdom, 1972

INDEX

E

F

G

H

I

K

L